Breaking Barriers

Breaking Barriers

100 personal accounts of mental ill health, recovery, and connection

edited by **Glenn Fosbraey** and **Katie Pether**

VP

Valley Press

First published in 2024 by Valley Press
Woodend, The Crescent, Scarborough, YO11 2PW
www.valleypressuk.com

ISBN 978-1-915606-25-9
Cat. no. VP0209

A CIP record for this book is available from the British Library.

Cover illustration by Rawpixel.
Cover and text design by Jamie McGarry.

Contents

Introduction

Lesley Black, Director of Student Support & Success, University of Winchester

I'm so delighted that you have chosen to read this wonderful anthology of texts. You will be taken on a journey that will open doors to some very personal stories; there are moments of despondency, moments of hope, but overall you will find, within this collection, the power of the individual spirit to create, to rise above, to speak from the wilderness and to share. Sharing our stories is an age-old tradition, it is part of what makes us human, creating our narratives through spoken or written artforms a form of truth-telling; it enables us to make sense of the things we experience and it allows us to learn from others – to understand the world from a different perspective. I hope that, through these writings, you find a deeper understanding of the worlds some of us live in, that you are spurred to find out more. But with this comes a caveat, within these pages you may encounter things that are challenging and distressing. Please take the time to look after yourself and seek support if you need it.

We all live with mental health and it's important that we treat it as seriously as we do our physical health. Each year around 1 in 4 people will experience some kind of mental health problem. If you are concerned for your own, or someone else's mental health, please seek support. Talk to someone you trust, your GP can be a good first port of call, as is the NHS 111 service in the UK. The Samaritans are available 24 hours a day, 365 days a year, and organisations like Mind offer information, advice and support.

For now, pull up a comfy chair and settle into this extraordinary collection of voices.

A note from the editors

This book contains personal accounts on the subjects of mental health and mental ill health from contributors aged between 18 and 83, male, female, transgender, and non-binary, from the UK, USA, Africa, and mainland Europe, and from a diverse range of ethnic backgrounds and occupations. In this way, we aim to show that mental health and mental ill health can impact upon everyone, regardless of age, ethnicity, gender, location, or occupation.

Reading about mental ill health in such a personal way may be a new experience for you, but it underlines the purpose of why we wanted to create this collection: to help create a society where people feel able to share what they are experiencing, even if it's difficult to say it out loud.

Content warning

We want you to look after your own psychological and personal safety, so we have included list of some mental health services available in the UK.

Please note this book will cover themes of suicide, self-harm, abuse, depression, anxiety, isolation, addiction, loss, eating disorders, OCD, and also contains some sexual references and strong language. The pieces shared in this book are personal accounts and therefore specific to individual authors and their own experiences. We encourage everybody to seek the right support for them.

If you're reading this and feeling up to it, do check in with those closest to you, as they may be struggling. If you're reading this and you *are* suffering with mental ill health, hopefully this book will show you that you're not alone.

Thank you for reading this, and in doing so being part of a society that is breaking barriers around the subject of mental health.

Glenn Fosbraey and Katie Pether

Support services

Anxiety UK

Charity providing support if you have been diagnosed with an anxiety condition.

Telephone: 03444 775 774 (Monday to Friday, 9.30am to 5.30pm)

Website: www.anxietyuk.org.uk

Bipolar UK

A charity helping people living with manic depression or bipolar disorder.

Website: www.bipolaruk.org.uk

CALM

CALM is the Campaign Against Living Miserably, for men aged 15 to 35.

Telephone: 0800 58 58 58 (daily, 5pm to midnight)

Website: www.thecalmzone.net

Men's Health Forum

24/7 stress support for men by text, chat and email.

Website: www.menshealthforum.org.uk/beatstress.uk

Mental Health Foundation

Provides information and support for anyone with mental health problems or learning disabilities.

Website: www.mentalhealth.org.uk

Mind

Promotes the views and needs of people with mental health problems.

Telephone: 0300 123 3393 (Monday to Friday, 9am to 6pm)

Website: www.mind.org.uk

No Panic

Voluntary charity offering support for sufferers of panic attacks and obsessive compulsive disorder (OCD). Offers a course to help overcome your phobia or OCD.

Telephone: 0844 967 4848 (daily, 10am to 10pm). Calls cost 5p per minute plus your phone provider's Access Charge

Website: www.nopanic.org.uk

OCD Action

Support for people with OCD. Includes information on treatment and online resources.

Telephone: 0845 390 6232 (Monday to Friday, 9.30am to 5pm). Calls cost 5p per minute plus your phone provider's Access Charge

Website: www.ocdaction.org.uk

OCD UK

A charity run by people with OCD, for people with OCD. Includes facts, news and treatments.

Telephone: 0333 212 7890 (Monday to Friday, 9am to 5pm)

Website: www.ocduk.org

PAPYRUS

Young suicide prevention society.

Telephone: HOPElineUK 0800 068 4141 (9am to midnight, every day of the year)

Website: www.papyrus-uk.org

Rethink Mental Illness

Support and advice for people living with mental illness.

Telephone: 0300 5000 927 (Monday to Friday, 9.30am to 4pm)

Website: www.rethink.org

Samaritans

Confidential support for people experiencing feelings of distress or despair.

Telephone: 116 123 (free 24-hour helpline)

Website: www.samaritans.org

SANE

Emotional support, information and guidance for people affected by mental illness, their families and carers.

Textcare: comfort and care via text message, sent when the person needs it most: www.sane.org.uk/textcare

Peer support forum: www.sane.org.uk/supportforum

Website: www.sane.org.uk/support

YoungMinds

Information on child and adolescent mental health. Services for parents and professionals.

Telephone: Parents' helpline 0808 802 5544 (Monday to Friday, 9.30am to 4pm)

Website: www.youngminds.org.uk

Abuse (child, sexual, domestic violence)

NSPCC

Children's charity dedicated to ending child abuse and child cruelty.

Telephone: 0800 1111 for children (24-hour helpline) 0808 800 5000 for adults concerned about a child (24-hour helpline)

Website: www.nspcc.org.uk

Refuge

Advice on dealing with domestic violence.

Telephone: 0808 2000 247 (24-hour helpline)

Website: www.refuge.org.uk

Alcoholics Anonymous

A free self-help group. Its '12 step' programme involves getting sober with the help of regular face-to-face and online support groups.

Telephone: 0800 917 7650 (24-hour helpline)

Website: www.alcoholics-anonymous.org.uk

Al-Anon

Al-Anon is a free self-help '12 step' group for anyone whose life is or has been affected by someone else's drinking.

Telephone: 0800 0086 811 (daily, 10am to 10pm)

Website: www.al-anonuk.org.uk

Drinkline

A free confidential helpline for people worried about their own or someone else's drinking.

Telephone: 0300 123 1110 (weekdays 9am to 8pm, weekends 11am to 4pm)

National Association for Children of Alcoholics

National Association for Children of Alcoholics offers free confidential advice and information to everyone affected by a parent's drinking including children, adults and professionals.

Telephone: 0800 358 3456 (Friday, Saturday and Monday 12pm to 7pm and Tuesday, Wednesday and Thursday 12pm to 9pm)

Website: www.nacoa.org.uk

SMART Recovery UK

SMART Recovery UK face-to-face and online groups help people decide whether they have a problem with alcohol and drugs, build up their motivation to change, and offer a set of proven tools and techniques to support recovery.

Telephone: 0330 053 6022 for general enquiries about SMART Recovery UK (9am to 5pm, Monday-Friday)

Website: smartrecovery.org.uk

Alzheimer's Society

Provides information on dementia, including factsheets and helplines.

Telephone: 0300 222 1122 (Monday to Friday, 9am to 5pm and 10am to 4pm on weekends)

Website: www.alzheimers.org.uk

Cruse Bereavement Care

Telephone: 0808 808 1677 (Monday to Friday, 9am to 5pm)

Website: www.cruse.org.uk/home

Rape Crisis

To find your local services phone: 0808 802 9999 (daily, 12pm to 2.30pm and 7pm to 9.30pm)

Website: www.rapecrisis.org.uk

A love letter

Katie, Mental Health First Aid Instructor

I don't wear black
Because I fear wearing it at your funeral.

Instead, when I see you,
I dress in vivid colour,
I wear the hues of our memories.
I cover myself in the shades of the countries we have visited,
And the drinks and dreams we have chased.

When we are together and when we are apart,
I laugh at the things we have done, the absurd things we have
    said and the people we have kissed.
The happiest memories of crawls, midnight brawls and crying
    on the sofa at three in the morning.
A week doesn't pass without a love letter sent by WhatsApp,

The letters are always replied to with another and another,
Endless love is given, and nothing is expected in return.

If there is ever a moment where you feel that weight is getting
    too close to your chest – call.
Our love knows no bounds and a two hour drive at two A.M.
    will feel like two minutes.

I don't wear black and, in my head, you'll stay.

The Wallflower

Clare, Family Support Worker

C wrote love letters to the monsters under the bed
Made of papier-mâché barricades
And arranging bear bones into swords.

C was alive alive alive and they were dead.
Some inside the trinket box in the shape of an elephant
And the rest in the waste basket case, alone

C was always alone, picking roses from next door
And pressing them between pages of hardback books
Snapping the stalk in half and watching the sap ooze
Onto the words and smudging them, watching the ink run.

Check, one two

Daniel, musician

It takes me about twenty minutes to leave the house because I have to check every window, door, tap, light switch, plug socket numerous times before I feel ready to step out onto the other side of the door.

Once I am out, maybe at a film or a garden centre, I constantly panic that I have forgotten something and somehow something slipped through the net. Twenty minutes now isn't enough. In fact, the burglars have now walked in through the ajar door, popped a pizza into the already switched on oven and have decided when they're wrapped up with this particular burglary to leave the straighteners on, just for a laugh.

This started in my twenties. An inability to trust myself and to always expect the absolute worst. My glass isn't half empty, it's knocked over and has covered the floor in water. I know the back door is locked, I've checked it three times but somehow I get into my car... turn the engine on, have a moment, turn it off and then go back into my house and check it again, just in case.

Of course, it's locked. It's always locked.

My friend Tom gave me a valuable bit of advice. Tell yourself out loud that you're doing the check as you're doing it. I do this now. "I am turning off the light... the light is now switched off... I am checking the bathroom tap... the bathroom tap is off". That sorta thing. Try it if you like, it helps.

I'm a little better but I still worry. I'm beginning to think I'll always be this way. I fully expect the final words on my deathbed to be along the lines off "I've been a lucky man and lived a good life with some wonderful people. Oh but can you drive back to the flat and check the George Foreman is definitely off before I can relax and croak it, please?"

It's just one part of me and I'm working on it. But do me a favour, if you see me at a cinema or a garden centre maybe put your arms around me and tell me that it's off/locked/unplugged. Then at least if it isn't, after filling out the insurance papers and signing the line on the next property I'll be renting, I can proudly lift my head up high and say "well, I told you so."

I came, I saw, I –

Mazie, Sales

Water to drown in please with a silver spoon,
eyes for days and nights rolled into this shelled hollow.
Eruption echoes from my mouth as nothing follows nothing,
carving through my charred and chattered teeth,
faceless autumn and grinding into soil,
my bones re-breaking over fractured mind,
snapping at nothing regaining nothing weaker and stronger,
but different forces space between the cavity and the breath into
the ears.
Holes inside the skull as the self-slips into the river I eat with,
and swallow building blocks finding the caved-in to prop up
and I see.

How can I?

Shakerah, social work assistant

"How can I help?" you say.

Well, for starters you could climb into my brain and try to massage it like an emptying tube of toothpaste in the hopes of squeezing out some drops of serotonin? Or is that physically impossible?

"How can I help you?" you ask earnestly as you look at me wide eyed whilst you finish washing up the pots and pans after you've cooked us a healthy scrumptious meal. I look over at the pile of washing you put on and dried once you got home from work. "I hate to see you like this." You've already started putting the clothes away.

"How can I help you?" you say as you hand over the baby for me to dry and cuddle after you've done her whole bath time routine. "Is it me? am I doing something wrong?" as you organise our finances and tell me that I don't need to return to work until I'm mentally ready to and that you've arranged to pick up another shift to cover this.

"How can I help you?" as you mentally protect me from the venomous words your child's mother tries to spit at me. You take every word like a bullet in your back turning them into sweet nothings as you whisper in my ear "how can I help you?"

"How can I help you?" you say as we sit in A&E after I insisted you didn't come. You hold my hand tight as we try to crack jokes whilst I'm losing the baby we were so excited for only a few weeks back. It is what it is. I try and rationalise to myself and you. I'm fine, we're fine. There's nothing we can do.

"How can I…" how can I sit here and allow you to keep supporting our family whilst I just exist? Even on my darkest days your light will always shine through. How can I stop feeling like this? Who is looking after you? While you do everything to look after me?

Not every day is dark and with you those dark days are fleeting and sparse. You are not a replacement for antidepressants or therapy but an added bonus, an inspiration, a partner, serotonin in human form.

...not what you think

Julie, Teaching Assistant

I hear voices; no, it's not what you think.
Do-gooders, experts, family and friends;
Loud enough to drive me to drink –
Or worse.
It's all about you; how you feel, they say –
I get it; I understand; I feel your pain.
And for the record, here's another cliché –
Hashtag 'metoo'.
But now it's my voice I hear, silently shout,
Shut up; leave me be; go to Hell –
You're driving me out
Of my mind!
Hey, don't feel bad that you can't help.
Stay with me, heed my silence… be kind.

He lost his baby too

Rajveer, Governance, Standards and Control Lead

He may not say it, he may not show it, he just isn't programmed
    that way
But his heart is broken, and he too carries the grief, through
    every moment, of every day
He lost his baby too
He wipes away her tears, then when no-one's around he sheds
    his own
He'll grieve in his own way, in his own time and often, he'll
    grieve alone
He lost his baby too
He says he's ok, he's fine, keeping busy, just tired
As if creating that false pretense is an act to be admired
He lost his baby too
He'll try to be strong, because that's a rule of masculinity, right?
He doesn't know it's safe to show emotions, so he keeps them
    out of sight
He lost his baby too
He had envisioned a life with his child, visions that never came
He didn't physically carry their baby but, he carries this absence
    all the same
He lost his baby too
He'll go back to work, probably before his mind is in the right
    place
And people will think he's doing better because he's gone back
    but, that really isn't the case
He lost his baby too
He won't say if he's struggling and, "how is dad doing?" isn't
    something that people generally ask
He doesn't know how to respond so he hides behind his
    armour, hides behind his mask
He lost his baby too

He's become a master of hiding, he's perfected that disguise
But you'll see unspoken pain, if you look deep into his eyes
He lost his baby too
So to all the dads grieving, rest, take the time you need to take
What you feel is completely normal, you're safe, it's ok for you
   to break
You lost your baby too

Welcome to My Mind (it's hell in here)

Tasha, Copywriter

I cannot remember a time when I wasn't mentally ill.

Christ, don't put that. Bit depressing, isn't it?

But isn't that the whole point? To be honest?

Yeah, but there's honest and then there's *too* honest. Do you want people thinking you've been batshit crazy since you were nine?

Good point.

What I meant to say was, I am mentally ill, but it's okay.

"It's okay." Are you kidding me? It's not okay at all, you idiot! Don't you see? Nothing is okay, and you aren't either.

But everything feels pretty okay now. Apart from you banging on. Would you give it a rest for a change? I'm trying to write here. I've got a deadline to meet.

Nope. Never. I need to be here all the time to make you question absolutely everything. Otherwise what would happen to you?

Uh, I'd be *normal*?

No, you'd be *stupid.* For a start, you wouldn't know that your writing sucks and nobody wants to hear what you have to say. And your work colleagues? They laugh at you behind your back because you're the most boring one in the group. Oh, and you know that friend who left you on read? They secretly find you *super* annoying and couldn't be bothered to entertain you with a reply. Plus, you've put on a few pounds since you were 19. Should probably do something about that. Without me, you wouldn't know nearly half of these things. It's a good job I'm here, really.

What if those things aren't true?

What do you mean? Of course they're true. It's me who said them.

Good point.

What about if I start by saying this: I've made peace with my mental illness.

I haven't made peace with you though.

Brilliant. Thanks.

What? It's true. Oh, don't be like that. You're so sensitive. No wonder everybody hates you. Fucking crying all the time over nothing.

It's a wonder I don't cry more when I have to put up with you.

Don't be so ungrateful. I told you just now, it's a blessing that I'm here.

A blessing is not what I'd call it. I have to fight with you every single day. When will I be able to rest? When will I be able to break free from you?

Why on earth would you want to do that?

Because I crave contentment. I crave genuine connection with people without questioning my place in their life. You've pestered me practically my whole life, plaguing every thought I have. Every social interaction. Every act of love. Every compliment. Every message. You even choke me some days, sitting on my chest, restricting my breathing, sending pins and needles over my body. When will you pack it in? When will you make me feel like I'm enough?

…When you start acting like you are.

Okay. Good point.

And when you stop being an annoying, boring lump of flesh.

Are you fucking kidding me?

Treading Water

Amy, Writer

I won't join you in the depths of your despair,
Because good would that do?
Other than drag you down further
Drowning with you.
Instead,
take my hand
I'll pull you towards the light.
Let's tread water
through these dark days and nights
Until you're ready to swim
Ride the waves
Towards happier days
I'll never let you give in
We will rise together
Breathe deep
It's you and me
Forever.

George Roff

Rosie, Communications Manager

I'm so proud to be your sister, George
You were the kindest person I knew
Funny, thoughtful, and silly
Just to name a few
I can't believe I'll never see you again
Or hear your high-pitched laugh
Together we made a mini team
And you were the better half
I'd do anything to give you one last hug
One last kiss goodbye
You were the best big brother out there
so all I can do is cry
I'll try to remember the good times
When we were little and used to play
I'll cherish those memories forever now
I really wish you could stay
I'm so grateful for our years together
And for the bond we will always share
I have so much left to tell you, George
This is all just so unfair
I will miss you for the rest of my life
But I know you're not very far
You will always be my big brother, George
No matter where you are.

George Roff lost his life to suicide at aged 26. We remember him for his infectious laugh, playfulness, and kindness. A much-loved son, brother and friend. We will love and miss you, always.

The Classroom

Gill, Teaching Assistant

Peace and quiet before the storm

Breathe in; breathe out.

Students coming,
      Chattering, clattering, cackling
Breathe in; breathe out.

Classroom crumbling!

The door opens:

      Bang!

Silence shattered.

Helianthus

Nicole, Sales & Marketing Executive

It tied its laces around my feet, dug me like a peg
into the carpet.
pile consumed my ankles and climbed the steak,
to my hips, to my chest.
it trickled down my arm, tying bows with my
thumbs. nose up with yawning eyes,
the bulb was weak. it ate its way through my
veins.
I was picked by the waist.
from under the handmade blind, a patch of light
fell on the seersucker. I was placed there.
wool splattered on your scrubs and you dug your
feet like beetles into the mattress.
you turned my chin to the window. yellow
reflected on your cheeks
as my disks began to beat. It drained away with
the hum of your bottom lip.

Common misconceptions about depression

Ione, full-time mum

"Hopefully this will make you smile" "Hopefully this can help cheer you up" It's not that I have nothing in my life that makes me smile, I still remember how to smile, I still know how to be happy, it's just hard to stay that way. There's always something negative around the corner or in the shadows of my brain that mean I feel like I don't deserve to be happy. Or there's just so much other stuff weighing me down, a cute video of a cat or a baby just isn't enough to pull me away from the darkness. It's not your job to make me happy. It's my own, yes you can help but unfortunately it does take a lot more than something funny to bring me out of myself. 100% supportive. Don't get me wrong, support is amazing! You're happy when I'm happy, sad when I'm down and angry when I am. However, too much support can be just as damaging as nothing at all. By all means validate my feelings but don't take them further by feeling them on my behalf. I'm feeling before I'm doing, reacting before responding. I'm missing that step in between where I ask myself "is this worth it?" Help me whilst I'm reacting, soothe me, tell me it's gonna be alright but then help me flip it, help me ask myself is this really worth all the emotion I'm giving the situation? Ask me what I can do about it. Don't give me solutions, help me get there, let me have that victory. I need to re-train my brain; sometimes my reactions are not worth the situation and I know that so don't join in – that makes my brain subconsciously feel like it's okay to be that way. "Should you be taking those tablets?" Having already had a bout of depression and been on these tablets, I know the risks. My body is not producing enough serotonin. If you're low on iron, you take iron supplements, why should there be a stigma on antidepressants? Yes, there are risks but I don't take them lightly, I know what to look out for and in all honesty, they are only step 1 of the process. There are so many more aspects to depression that we are still discovering. On the flip side: the "just take tablets" response is just as bad. As I said earlier they are just one part of the process, I have to do some work to do too. "If you ever want to talk, I'm here" I do appreciate the notion, don't get me wrong. Talking is exhausting. I'm lucky this time around people close to me are very aware of what I'm going through and are doing their damndest to understand (sometimes a very difficult feat) however there's only so much talking one can do. When you talk to someone about it, you feel guilty. You're monopolizing the conversation, you know they feel bad for you. You worry that you're depressing them and stressing them out. Please don't offer to talk if you know you can't handle it. A better response is: Sorry to hear you're struggling, if you want to hang out and get away from it all you know where I am. I don't always want to talk about my depression, I give it too much power as it is!

Frost

Lucie, Assistant Stage Manager

The frost reveals something
Tracks footfall
Welcomes theories
The moon highlights
Casting shadows with her bright wand
Christmas is around the corner
What does that really mean?
A man dressed
Giving gifts
Taking payment in cookies and milk
I stand in her moonlight
Wondering this
Thinking I shouldn't be
So I go home, I cradle sadness
Crying itself to sleep
But hush now
Sadness has gone quiet
Eyes closed
Toes still
I always make it worse
So I stay quiet
Not to move
Not to startle
I add my footprints with the rest let the future historians
    decipher why
Simple answer
Though now I ponder this tree
Currently a seat for the strangers
Formerly a shade for the villagers
Planted as a gift
To sadness
Each year sprouted

Each tear watered
Each fruit nourished
The soil now littered
Once worshiped
I stand on holy ground I decide
Great things have happened and great things will
So Sadness does what she does best and smiles
waning again
Into the night
Long cries
And I stay still
For who am I to disturb?

Fragments

Cassie, Senior Teaching Associate

We know how this story will end.

We read to the end of each page and turn to the next, we have to keep going forwards. There is no putting the book down and walking away. There is no re-writing the future and no reading backwards. There is no cure, we can only slow its progression.

Forwards march.

Your stories are like pieces of a jigsaw except some of the pieces belong to other puzzles. They have had their corners bitten off and chewed so that they appear to fit, but gaps are still visible. Dad has become a puzzle master, a skilled player in the game. He views the fragments of a lifetime and helps you to narrate them, creating a picture from the pieces.

Language has become a slippery creature, wriggling and writhing on the page. Sentences are squashed, words missing, syllables pushed together to produce the right effect.

We all laughed. We thought it was with you, but it turned out to be a spelling error, unknown.

MUM:	Grass snakes in Scotland are armless
ME:	Ha! Good joke
BROTHER:	Haha! Very funny
MUM:	No this is for real
BROTHER:	I'm sure they are harmless, but they are also definitely *arm*less
MUM:	Grass snakes are armless, but adders are not

I don't know the right way to feel. It's a humour that carves a pit in my stomach. A laughter that claws and crawls its way from my heart to my stomach.

I don't remember the last time you asked about my day, my week, my work, my life. It sounds selfish, I know, but I miss our telephone calls and I miss talking to you about things, having you ask questions about me, and having you offer advice. The emptiness weighs heavily.

When we talk sometimes your eyes glaze over, seeing something I don't. I wait for you to return and come back to me. *As I was saying...*

Is that the time? It creeps up on you when your back is turned, snaps at your heels. It is a treacherous creature. I pause to enjoy a moment. I just need a second longer but I feel it's breath on my neck, its growing impatience. So we march forwards once more. With each step you become more fragmented. Another jigsaw piece missing, forgotten, lost.

MUM: Do you think I'll get better

DAD: I hope so

MUM: I've been trying really hard. Trying to think
          about things. Remember more.

Each day we are lucky that you are still you. You still laugh and sing, though the words are uncertain. You still enjoy silly games, crafting and painting. Those parts remain. They are the fragments we treasure and stitch back together.

As I Walked the Hyacinth Garden

Arthur, Actor

My silent life was real, like an oriole today,
My wandering sight was soft in love and willing to obey,
And I sensed in the reddening air what the poets of Babylon say.

"There is nothing but pleasure and pain, there is peacetime,
    there is war,
And we've travelled this burning carnelian road uncounted
    times before,
And we glimpse in one mortal moment the way of the heavenly
    law."

I was there, the oak was oaking, the larch was larching, the
    birch was birching,
And my heart was loudly humming – I was seeing without
    searching,
And I laughed because I saw a big fat blue jay by me perching!

I was free from gross desire to translate things I think,
For I could see the violet blaze and a dazzling bundle of pink,
And human concern for order, and my manic depression, could
    sink.

Around my life I felt no prodding inquiry or burden,
The world was fluid once again, but I knew that it must harden –
When I moved in Minneapolis, my soul was born in Jordan,
And no one needed words at all, as I walked the Hyacinth Garden.

The Haunted Man: Dickens and Mental Health

Emily, primary school teacher

I began research for this article sat by a twinkling Christmas tree with *The Muppets Christmas Carol* blaring from the television. In all honesty, when thinking about mental health and watching the Muppets my first thought was the puppets themselves. Miss Piggy with an extreme infatuation with herself, Beaker with his crippling anxiety, The Count with his obsessive counting and I don't have the time nor energy to begin thinking about Animal or Oscar the Grouch. So, I'll start again... after sitting for a long time concerned about the Muppets, I then began to think about Charles Dickens. Now, that is a man who knows how to write about sorrow. Almost too well.

Charles John Huffam Dickens is a name familiar to everyone. His impact on literature is immense but what I was not aware of was his influence on society in bleak Victorian England. By his early 30's, Charles Dickens was the guy that everyone wanted to know. He was rich, young, intelligent and seemed to have it all. However, an awfully difficult childhood filled with struggle sent him on the path to depression. His friends often quoted that his depression worsened when he was writing a new novel. The weight of expectation for each novel to be better than the last, more entertaining, and more impactful was too much of an ordeal. This sense of mania would be the fuel that propelled him to finish each novel. Naturally, the book would be a huge success and the cycle would continue. He was trapped, by himself, in glory. This same depression would plague him for his entire life until old age, where it would finally suffocate his creativity.

This mania did have a way of seeping into his work and some of his many characters were haunted by mental illnesses. For example, in the book *Great Expectations,* Arthur Havisham suffered from "the horrors" which modern-day doctors have equated to alcohol withdrawal. Furthermore, Dickens also had a way of expressing physical medical ailments in his work long before they were officially recognised by doctors of the time. He challenged medicine by writing about learning difficulties that, although common today, were not known in Victorian England. As seen in this quote from *Bleak Street* when describing the shopkeeper, "He can make all the letters separately and he knows most of them separately when he sees them… but he can't put them together." Some have theorised that this may be the first written description of dyslexia – made more impressive because *Bleak Street* was published thirty years before the term itself reached medical literature.

Besides his brilliant and cherished tales, Dickens became a social reformer. He was a key player in the development of homeless shelters for women and the first pediatric hospital in the United Kingdom. Although haunted by his own struggles with depression, Charles Dickens' impact on society cannot be overshadowed.

"No one is useless in this world who lightens the burdens of another."

The Demon on My Back

Kieran, Charity Director

This train will be calling at: Newton Abbot

I stand at the edge of the platform, waiting for the right time. It's strange how everything that led up to this moment comes to me now. It's almost as if my brain knows what's coming. The death of my grandma, my whole family sitting in a church pew, gazing up at a giant depiction of the crucifiction. That was the first day I felt it, the demon crawling up my back in a place where demons shouldn't be able to enter.

Totnes

Wherever I went, it clung. My work, where I was once relatively happy, now I started to hate everything and everyone there. All at once I felt as if my friends were laughing at me behind my back, pretending to care about me, secretly plotting how they could ostracise and belittle me.

Exeter St Davids

And as the weeks and months went on, the demon's grip grew steadily tighter, its long black limbs crawling over my shoulders and around my neck, choking the life out of me. Alone in my bed it would whisper things to me, telling me how I had no use to anyone, how in fact, I was a burden to those around me, how in reality it had always been that day even before it had arrived.

Taunton

They say that if you are told something enough times you will eventually believe it, maybe that's true. The weird thing is that the demon that I had once thought was the root of all my problems started to become the only one I could trust. That choking feeling became warm and comforting, like a nice scarf you get from your grandma at Christmas when you are a kid. The things it told me were exactly the things I needed to hear. I just needed to be alone, just needed to stay inside for a bit longer.

Reading

One night, my mum called me to tell me my grandad had died. I told her what I thought she wanted to hear, secretly thinking that this made sense. I went into the bathroom. The demon pushed me forward, it lifted my razor to my wrist.

London Paddington

Even now the demon is here, telling me this is a mistake, telling me that this will just make things worse. All that will come is more judgement, more mocking laughter. But my mum and dad are on either side of me, the train doors have opened and waiting for the right time to get on, I'm going to see a therapist. He says that lots of people have a demon on their back like me, and that whatever it's telling me is wrong. I get on the train and sit and as the Devon countryside passes I feel that, for the first time in months, maybe just maybe, the demon's grip has loosened a little.

The weight of my hair

Susmita, writer

is most felt when it comes away
so easily. I stand in the shower, clutching at clumps –
like seaweed waving, sweeping
along the ocean floor.

I know the freedom of running my fingers
over smooth, prickled scalp. It misses my mother's
fingers gently rubbing my hair with
hibiscus scented oil. Her weekly routine
to ensure a mass of midnight blue curls
has come to nothing.

Now it's just a rash of skin
protected by a silk scarf.

First published in Rough Diamond Poetry, October 2021.

The Final Fall

Dan, Refuse Collector

Silent night, lonely life
All round me right now is quiet
Only I can hold the light
Only I can stall the riot

The crazy sprawl has grown so tall
And I can't keep control no more
The final fall to end it all
Has never been so close before

The lowing dim is closing in
The faster flow into the brink
It's ruining my everything
And made a mess of what I think

Words upon words

Samara, Quality Assurance Team Leader

Constantly tired putting on a front that everything is okay, and you are happy.

Continuously surrounded by family and friends and their love and support, but with moments that whilst you are surrounded you feel alone.

Self-doubt, shame and thinking the worst of yourself.

Wanting to achieve more, knowing you can achieve more but a voice in the back of your head constantly whispering that you are just not good enough.

Continuing to push forward because there are days that you love yourself and who you are. Not every day is dark and lonely, but some days are bright and filled with pockets of happiness and joy.

The Knot

Naomi, Student Advisor

The Knot lives inside my body.
I think it has done for all my life,
And will remain there: an alternate organ,
A spherical tangle in my core, the middle of me.

Sometimes I barely know that it is there –
It is slack and floats quietly and calmly,
Anchoring me, keeping me balanced.
I can acknowledge it, appreciate it, live with it.

Sometimes its strings start to gently pull,
Binding the ball together, reminding me politely of its existence.
The gaps between the threads close in,
But with still enough space to breathe.

Sometimes all I can feel is The Knot.
The strings have been yanked and the sphere is tense, muddled,
    hard.
It no longer floats but is stuck, rooted:
It becomes me, and I become it.
But I know now that it will not stay like this forever.
Whether it takes hours, or days, or weeks, or months,
It will loosen.

The Knot will not define me.

It's hard to explain

Josie, Events Manager

It's hard to explain
As I don't really account it to
Anything specific
That's going on in my life
As I'm pretty happy

A feeling of overwhelmingness not related to anything
That can bring me into a panicked state
Or one day an extreme low for no reason at all.

I needed rest

Sandra, Civil Servant

It's like trying to land two planes at one time
You know at some point one of the planes has to crash eventually

Vulcan Sundered

PumpkynVine, writer

You cannot be as you were before
Not when your core has been obliterated
All that made you poured through the fissures
Catching up every paper piece of you
Blistering your heart
Till you are gasping on the ragged ashes
Of memories that once tasted sweet as spring rain
Of smiles stabbed through with needle and thread, twisted and
   misshapen now
Of dreams disintegrated on stunned fingertips
Yet reaching out for stardust

You cannot be as you were before
She's not there anymore
The storm's brittle malice laughs
Lingers on the echoes of destruction
In the hollows left behind
I know you're cold
The tattered remnants of your mind trying to find some rhyme
   or reason
But there is none
None of us are owed that illusive delight

You cannot be as you were before
So stop
Can't you see? Your broken bleeding nails scrapping at her grave
The endless scream you hide behind *I'm fine* as silent as her
   death
That ocean churning just past sight
The dams won't hold forever
So darling
Just stop

You cannot be as you were before
And that's ok
We've lingered here long enough, don't you think?
Let them go, all those fragmented, piercing slivers you clutch to
Thinking the air will drift from your lungs should you loose
　　your grip
Yet every breath presses against their jagged edges
Cutting you
Choking you
So let them go

You cannot be as you were before
But you can yet bloom
Curled and sniffling raw little mite
Feel the whispering tendrils coaxing saplings from all that was
　　before
Damp and soft now
You press your cheek into its warmth
Scarred tears soaked and salty
Tentative leaves yet furled, peeking at a faded misty sun

You cannot be as you were before
But do not let that hardened shell cocoon all that could be
Do not let reverberations of potent trembling fear thunder
　　down your spine
Shaking new foundations
Do not let scythes swung by others reap that which has hardly
　　even been sawn
And do not drizzle poison on those fragile roots, shyly mating
　　with your tender soil

You cannot be as you were before
So accept who flourishes in her place
For she has weathered all forces of nature bottled up inside her
    shivering soul
Unstoppable and brutish in their merciless war
She needs a hand, a moment to catch her breath
Give her a blanket, some cake and a cup of tea
Listen till the turmoil's tranquil
As crumbs fall from her chin and steam curls up her nose

You cannot be as you were before
And isn't that magnificent?
A whole new you stands in its wake
Thicker as a tree grows rings with each passing year
Bark under your palm so warm to touch in dappled steady
    sunlight
Bright leaves brush against your upturned fluttering lashes

You cannot be as you were before
So smile darling
And take a step
And the next
And the one after that
Till you too marvel at all the footprints you have left behind

You cannot be as you were before
But wouldn't she be proud to see how far her footsteps stretch
    into a new horizon?

A Lifetime

Malee, US Student

Raise your hand if you are…

an overthinker who
is…
Searching endlessly, wandering endlessly, questioning endlessly
for a lifetime to call your own?

Because you were taught about others but never about yourself?

Do you think…

Laughter can shorten a lifeti— and tears can make it longer?

How many lives are born and

passed

within one's lifetime?

How does one even measure a lifetime?

*In seconds, minutes, hours, days, tears, laughter, heartbeat, or
regrets?*

Finding my way

Paddy, Assistant Editor

Sometimes it's as simple as not wanting to get out of bed for the day.

Other times it's harder, like being on a ship drifting in the sea. Isolated and alone.

It's as though there's a dark cloud drifting just above your head, but you feel like it has its own weight, pushing you down and keeping you still.

You're not quite sure if you'll ever see the sunlight. Everything's blocked out and you're engulfed in shadow.

But then it manifests. Pushing down on your chest. You can feel the tightness and pressure as if there was a storm coming.

You can barely move or speak, you can hardly find the strength to stand.

Your heart beats fast and slow, you panic and think you're on the edge of living. The existential dread becomes the dominant sensation you can feel, even to your bones. Your eyes look heavy, anyone would think you haven't slept in days.

Nothing seems like it'll ever be good again.

You spiral into a vast pit of nothingness where you only have intrusive thoughts and the sense of shame you've been living with for your formative years.

It's like standing in a forest and not being able to see the sky through the branches and leaves. You know it's there but there's no conceivable way to escape the shadow.

You put on a brave face, smile and laugh and pretend like everything's fine. Never letting anyone know that you feel hollow on the inside. Even though you know your friends and family care about you, you can't say a word because you're worried about how they'll react.

So you hide away, draw the curtains and ignore the world around you. Internalise all of your feelings and blame yourself for every experience you've ever had in your life.

As much as you try, you cannot sleep. Your emotions are pushing you and acting as caffeine. Being able to settle and calm yourself is beyond your capacity, so you lie there, barely able to breathe.

Unfortunately, you try and cope through unhealthy means. You drink, you smoke and just try and hide it all away. You just don't know how to manage the constant battle that's raging inside of yourself.

You can find ways to deal with it. Although it may be scary and you feel like you're treading water, you have the power to push through. Sharing your feelings is the first step you can take.

Think of it like a light switch. You've tried to walk through the hallway in the dark all of your life and assume you know where to go. You've stubbed your toe, knocked into a radiator, you've continued anyway. Then you find the switch. You can reach it. You can illuminate your path and find your way, even though you'd never felt like that before.

And there it is, a way to try and feel like yourself again. No matter how fleeting the feeling is, you know it's there.

Life doesn't seem as dark.

Doesn't everyone do that?

Sophie, Digital Marketing Manager

I've always assumed everyone's inner monologue was as vengeful as mine.

If you don't make it to that lamppost before that passing car, something bad is going to happen today. If I really pick up the pace I can make it there first.

You didn't turn your straighteners off now your flat's going to burn down and everyone will be trapped inside. I'll just tell everyone I've forgotten my purse so I can go back and check.

You didn't lock the front door, now someone's inside waiting for you to come back. I've only really just joined the M4, I can go back and check.

She's waiting to tell me, to remind me and I can't trust myself and my own memory. Was that today? Do I remember turning them off or was that yesterday? It will consume me. I'll just go and double check. Hob: off. Straighteners: off. Windows: closed. Door: locked.

It's all there, I can go to bed.

You're going to die and that's it.

There's nothing else for you to do or see or be a part of. No more friends, no more family, no more adventures, nothing left to experience. Try and picture it. The absolute nothingness. I dare you.

Are you doing it right? Your life. What's the point, right? What's the point in anything you're doing?

I can't breathe.

I'm crying in a completely new way and my body doesn't know what to do. I've thrown off the covers, I'm on my hands and knees on the floor. I need to make it to the bathroom because I'm going to vomit. I'm dry heaving and dry heaving. Convulsing through sobs and sweating thinking about what it's like to no longer exist.

I'm lying on the linoleum of my bathroom floor and I peel my shoulder out from under me and walk back to bed.

But, doesn't everyone do that?

Everything Is Going To Be Alright

Claire, poet

I've always been considered quite bright
this has not helped me quiet the waterfall
of disappointed faces roaring with reasons
for not following through on their part of a bargain

I'm a foolish negotiator paying in advance
with interest a trusting cynic believing words
those three magic words came first
'*In the beginning*' but who's narrating?

If I climb the falls and follow the river South
to the source of potential, I'll still be alone
with an urge to jump into the open mouths
bubbling up from hungry ground

I'm getting worse, loud and repetitive noises hurt
like boiling brain scold, like stubbing all my memories
perhaps I'm becoming pre-cycled glass
crashing into yawning blue plastic

I'm a fool and anger lives in my skin
like red geraniums boasting domestic bliss
from a UPVC window ledge
perhaps I'm a bag-for-life with a hole in

If I seek wisdom I hide in the cave behind the falls
sweeping a flaming torch across unpainted walls
searching corners for a Hermit to become
with a pet spark in a jar

I consider myself a lost tourist
without a map or language
trying to navigate by reading runes in eyes
perhaps I'm a creatrix witnessing being seen

Or a fool chasing their own tale
there's no avoiding it
the leap of faith
diving blind into dark waters

If I float naked at night in this pool
a flesh of questions surfacing
overwhelmed by starlight
I'll unlock the moon and count distance as a friend.

Borrowed Time

CJ, writer

Tonight's the night.

That's what I've whispered to myself before bed for nearly a decade, or much rather, the raging shadow inside me has – my impersonator, puppet master, and oldest but not dearest of friends: my depression. This enigmatic entity resides comfortably in the furthest recesses of dark matter, using its boundless influence to corrupt my mind, blacken my heart, and poison my soul. Usually around now, as the waking world is swallowed by black, silence and cold, seeming so afar, so indifferent to the burdens of one mere man in his own pocket of universe, it stirs from its pretend slumber and comes out to play…

…and here it is. Right on cue.

Knock, knock, knock.

Equilibrium is now a distant memory.

Listening to rain sputtering against glass, I contemplate a solitary candle wavering low, desperately hoping the habitual blend of cannabis, mirtazapine and quetiapine will send me to oblivion before my own hand does. Forever. As my eyelids turn heavier, head lighter, I wonder how it would be once the remaining grains of sand empty from the hourglass, to have my lungs draw their last breath, mind conjure its final thoughts and trickeries, heart perform its closing beat, to know I would stop being Charlie shortly, only to become flesh and bone, a blip vanishing as quickly as it appeared.

Did you take 3 tablets or all of them?

Memories bob on the surface of my consciousness.

I feel Mum's bronze arms wrapped around me, the Floridian sunlight beating down upon us through Cinderella's Castle while I clutch my clown duck soft toy and sip on a Ribena carton.

I gaze across the table at Prezzo to Jasmin on our first date, to her ethereal, arresting brown eyes, the clusters of freckles on her inner cheeks, and her sublime tresses of straight chestnut hair, curious as to whether angels really do walk among us, casting light on all that is dark, warmth on all that is cold. I run my hands through the thick coat of my yellow Labrador, Preston, feeling the air press against me as he waggles his tail like a propeller. I see Nan; not how she was in the hospice with her body and spirit starved from terminal cancer, but in the heart of the New Forest alongside her two retrievers, with a tuft of brown hair sitting atop her head, colour permeating her face, and a beam dancing gently across her lips as if she was listening to Elvis for the first time. I hear Gran sharing anecdotes of her astonishing 104-year existence, spanning across world wars, recessions, numerous prime ministers and shifting realities, meanwhile the papery touch of her fingers traces across my tiny untainted hands. I remember my father joining me briefly in the lounge to play with my Thomas the Tank Engine set – the only time I recall him doing such a thing. Wherever he is now, whoever he is, whatever he's doing, I vaguely hope somewhere, deep down, he's proud of me, and knows I don't blame him for this.

I don't blame anyone but myself.

That's the way it is.

Beyond these recollections, on the other side of the dark waters, pansies flutter to the wailing winds, colossal waves crash down upon the shores of past, present and future, and a drone hangs in the air like every baby hummingbird in the world were all taking their first flight at once. I see everyone I've ever known, or thought I knew, stood shoulder-to-shoulder as far as my eyes can see: the good, the bad, the beautiful and the ugly. Every girl I've ever loved.

Every disapproving teacher after my teenage self misbehaved. Every therapist studying me with their inquisitive stares. Every bully who found reassurance by agonising me instead of looking deeper into themselves. Every stranger whose path entangled with mine at one point or another.

Tick, tick, tick.

I reminisce about all I've achieved in the 9719 days that I've walked the earth: landing a lead role in the Robin Hood play at primary school, receiving my GCSE and A-Level results, writing a novel at the age of 19, passing my driving test with one minor, donning my mortarboard hat and gown and graduating with First Class Honours beneath the slanted roof of Winchester Cathedral, the final resting place of Jane Austen nearby.

Then I suddenly realise none of it matters, for all roads lead to this same place, this same moment – the final act. People have always told me there's light at the end of the tunnel, but I've spent so long as a remnant of my former self, drifting through limbo aimlessly, that when I eventually emerge, it will only be to step out into an eternal night, where one doesn't live but merely exists on borrowed time, contending against the tides of fate by delaying the inevitable, all the while bearing the great weight of a false smile.

Wind at my back, content in my heart, I stand at the edge of the world, peering into the bottomless abyss, ready to be cradled in your arms and delivered into the far beyond of nothingness – paradise. Do not feel sorrow now, for when I cross this bridge and slip away soundlessly into space and time, know flowers will keep on growing, the sun continue shining, and the world, in all its mysteries and wonders, will carry on, just as it always has, just as it always will.

Bells begin to toll above the clouds.

So be it.

I take a quick bow and step off the brink unhesitatingly. Going…
going –

Gone.

The alarm jolts me from sleep. I lay staring at the ceiling, beyond it, tears cascading down my face silently, before forcing myself to get up. I open the bedside drawer to see my tablets are still in their packets.

If you can't live for yourself, then you must live for others.

Still dazed, dread hanging over me every step, every breath, I stagger into work.

"How are you?" a colleague says.

Burdened by regrets of the past, worry for the future, and condemnation for the present.

"I'm fine. Thanks for asking," I reply.

Progress

AR, Medical Admin

progress isn't linear
i repeat this like a mantra
hoping that it would sink into my mind
like those words from years before
i want them to be true.
but why do i keep coming back to the same place?
same memories and compulsions and…
progress isn't linear
it follows a curve
highs and lows that theme park designers could only dream
keep the giga coasters
i've gotten more adrenaline from sitting in bed.
i repeat the words again
knowing if it were anyone else i would be saying sweet words
kind and understanding
but i'm rubber and there is no glue
everything bounces off me and falls back to bounce off and falls
    back to bounce off.
progress is a story from quentin tarantino
you watch the scenes go and go and return back to the familiar
    places, familiar people
from a different angle
with hindsight.
overlaps and relapse
evidence of the cruel curvature of progress
resources and resistance prove i am not the same
and yet…
knowledge helps to arm against the curve
threatening to become a pleat
it pushes it back with a support for the progress to only fold
    into an obtuse angle
but it's not lost.
progress isn't linear
but i know i'm getting better.

Don't Interrupt My Today

Jack, Actor

I'm trying to write inside the oh-so-beautiful-not-full-of-itself
  café.
Always a cafe.
I dunno.
It's like some Portaloo to the past:
the mysterious cellar door into the mind's what's-it-called.
New memories painting over
like a vandalised headstone.
This café, same building mum bought ornaments
and shit furniture when it used to be
"the place"
to buy ornaments and shit furniture.
And I "need to go find a job," she'd tell me.

In one ear, tumble-weeding out the other.

Don't really know what I'm talking about half the time.
Lately, I've been giving my despicable thoughts some context.
Save my eyeballs puking into pillowcases again.

The café's owner asked if she minded singing to me.
I said, everything's white noise these days, and my brain likes
  that.
She then gave me some cake.

Devotion

Dawson, US student

I, confused on the definition of 'Greed'
  perplexed by the justification of 'Need'
  a has-been seeking time-travel
  who realized the past is the past

I, unfurling anxious wings
  scared to fly from the nest

I, a hopeless knight in shining armor,
  crusading for his own voice
  marching home after defeat

I, who loved stuffed animals as a kid,
  a teddy with a fuck-ton of stitches
  short on thread for his needle

I, praying for forlorn sleep
  staring into bags under my eyes,
  holes widening in my memory

I, devoted to a distant star
  warmed by her blazing heart,
  introduced to color once more

I, begging again for her smile,
  throwing words into a black veil
  in denial of our disconnection,
  blind to the cracks in my reality

I, apologizing to shadows of her,
  showing penance for her,
  brandishing knives for her,
  digging in deep for her.

I, her fool and follower.

Do You See Me?

Sarah, Music Therapy Group

Do you see me crying in the rain?
Do you hear me screaming in the storm?
Do you see the pain in my eyes?
Do you feel the sadness behind my smile?

When I'm silent, can you hear me
Calling out to you?
When I'm anxious,
Do you see my fear?

When I am angry do you ask me why?
When I run, do you follow me?
When I panic, will you calm me?
When I need time, will you be kind?

When I am overwhelmed,
Can you reassure me?

Do I scare you when I – lose control?

Do I upset you when – I talk out of turn?
Do I let you down when – I don't turn up?
Do I offend you when – I don't reply?

Will you look beyond my mask?
...Do you see me?
I'm still here,
In front of you,

Fighting in my mind.
The story of my life.
Will you be my friend...
...And sit with me

       And just let me...
          ...Be me.

You are as good as anybody else

Mollie, Entertainment Journalist

A golden shovel, after Mary Shelley's Frankenstein

I start with stacks of paper as thick as an arm. *The*
stark sheets, once spread, pave a path to a hidden *world*.
When the author licked his pen nib, added colour *to*
jargon, stitched serifs with spiderwebs, he flecked *me*
and put freckles on a face I'd grown tired of. I *was*
a bud born mistaken for a thorn. If doctors ask to see *a*
hole, I fuel them with letters; they won't see the *secret*
life squeezed between lines, a lemon juice cipher *which*
glows under fire. I am the ash relearning ember. *I*
am a corpse learning to run. When young I *desired*
a plastic patient wristband *to*
label every limb. Now I know my name is *divine*.

The
hidden

face   I was
born
with

glows   I am
learning

my name

The Long Walk

Donna, Secondary school teacher

Mile 1, we're happy chatting. 'Putting the world to rights' we call it. Others maybe would call it a bitch and a moan. But it's healthy to vent. Always so much to moan about in this life. Mile 3, we're chatting about the future, hopes and aspirations, and things that are coming up. Mile 5, we talk about family and other friends and things that are going on with them. Things are fine. We are laughing and taking the mickey out of each other. But then it stops. Silence. The pace quickens. What happened? Things were fine and normal. By mile 8, I just want to get home; this walk has become a test of endurance both physically and mentally and it's exhausting. I don't understand why things have changed.

I think back over the conversations we have just had, what did I say wrong? I find nothing. But then, we've been here before and the pattern is always the same. There will be something that I've said that, to me, was nothing or a meaningless throw away comment, but it's something that you have latched on to and it's growing in your head like a garden weed smothering out all other thoughts. I ask if you are okay, you say you are fine. I ask what did I do / say? and you say nothing. You are fine. All is well. You don't know why I might think there is something wrong.

We walk on. My legs ache and my feet ache,, but my head hurts the most. It is swinging between confusion, frustration and anger. This irrationalness makes me angry. But I try to be fair. You don't mean it. You're not well. But it is so hard. I kind of want to shout at you because my life is falling apart and yours isn't and yet you are the one storming on ahead, crying and not talking. It is a bright sunny day, and yet the weight of the black storm clouds surrounding us is suffocating and I don't want to be here. But I want to make sure that you are ok because, despite this moment, I care and I love you and I want my bright, funny, mile 1-5 friend back.

I watch your body swaying in the distance as you walk at a pace that I cannot match. I don't know how to reach out to you and yet there is nothing more that I want to do. But I also want to leave you there and go home. I was never good at riddles and problem-puzzles, and the puzzle that is you is one that I do not even know where to begin. You're making my head hurt.

We arrive home. You go straight to your room and start crying. Your partner goes to comfort you. I have a drink, sit at the table and am still unsure what happened. What did I do? Finally, you come down, we hug. We make dinner. Till next time.

Present Perfect Continuous

Alanna, EFL Teacher

Okay, guys, we're going to review the present perfect continuous tense today. Remind me, how do we make the present perfect continuous tense?

Good, *subject + have* or *has + been + verb-ing*. And the negative?

That's right, *subject + haven't* or *hasn't + been + verb-ing*. Well remembered.

Now, look at the sentence on the board: "I have been feeling sad lately." How do we use this tense? Am I still feeling sad now?

I am, yes. Very good. And is this starting now?

No, it's not, you're right. When did it start?

In the past, yes. Do we know how long in the past? When did this action start?

Well, which word tells us about the time?

"Lately," good. So, when is "lately?" When does "lately" start?

Not quite. Longer than a couple of hours. Any other ideas?

Maybe a few days, maybe a week, maybe a few weeks. Okay good, that's one way we can use present perfect continuous. What about this example: "she has been crying." Is she still crying now?

Maybe, yes. But could it mean something else?

Yes, that's right. Maybe she stopped a very short time ago. How do we know if someone has been crying?

Their eyes are red, yes.

Good, their face is wet.

They look sad, absolutely. So, we can see the result of the action. We can see after the action. Well done, guys. Okay, now let's compare the present perfect continuous with the present perfect simple. Look at these two examples: "I haven't slept" and "I haven't been sleeping." Do these two sentences mean the same?

Not quite. What's the difference between these two? Look at the first sentence, "I haven't slept." When didn't I sleep?

Last night, okay. Only last night? Or, how many nights?

Good, just one. I'm talking about one action; a finished action sometime in the past. Do we know when?

Recently. Probably last night.

What about the second sentence: "I haven't been sleeping." How many nights?

More than one. Maybe 2, 3, 4 nights. Maybe a week. Maybe a month. Very good, guys. And is this just starting now?

No, it isn't. It started in the past and it has continued until now. Look at me, can you tell? Can you see it?

Oh, stop it. You're very sweet. Okay, so do we know when it started?

Yes, you're right. Three weeks ago. Well remembered. And what do I add when I want to say how long something happened for?

Do you remember? I just said it.

Good, "I haven't been sleeping *for* three weeks." Wonderful. What if I want to tell you the time that something started? Which word do I use then?

"Since." Fantastic. Can I say "I haven't been sleeping *since* three weeks?"

No, you're right. So, if I'm talking about when something started, what could I say? "I haven't been sleeping since…"

Good, "since November 10th, for example."

"Since the days got shorter," yes, we can also reference a past action with "since."

Absolutely, "since I stopped taking my meds." Excellent work, guys.

What was that?

Yes, of course. I'm fine.

Why do you ask?

Reframing

Lesley, University Director

I sit in the empty car park,
staring unseeing through the blurred window.
Rain makes a kaleidoscope of the view,
tears fracture yet more the altered image.
I catch a glimpse of my grey face
reflecting the sky and space I am in.
What was is gone.
What might have been will never be known.
A new picture will emerge from the shattered image.

The Imposter

Sam, Secondary School Teacher

The subtlest evils are often the most destructive. The malicious little voice in your ear. The imposter.

It whispers at first. Just loud enough for you to notice. You brush it off, you pretend it isn't there. But the second you begin to hear its vicious lies, it has you. You've acknowledged it. Then it has power; power that it can wield over you. Once it realises it has the slightest grip, it starts to claw its way into your head, further and further until it can properly dig its claws in, not caring what it destroys in its attempt to keep its control over you.

I used to think I could ignore it.

As a writer, I'm fortunate enough to be able to say I've had successes in my career. I've written for television channels, written articles for websites, even been published in a creative anthology. It's my biggest passion; the thing I pour my heart and soul into.

"Who would want to read this?" says the imposter. "Don't you feel embarrassed? The arrogance you must have to think this is worth anything to anyone." Its grip slowly tightens.

At the end of the Covid-19 pandemic, I stumbled on a new career path, and I began my training to become an English teacher. I've been blown away by the support and encouragement of everyone I've worked with, and now in my first year as a fully qualified teacher, I am settling into a routine and beginning to build meaningful relationships with staff and students.

"What an awful job you're doing," says the imposter. "It's not enough to be a disappointment in your own life, now you've decided to jeopardise the lives of innocent children too?" Its grip slowly tightens.

Just over a year ago, I met a woman who has become the love of my life. She is everything I could have ever asked for: kind, funny, beautiful, passionate, and encourages me every day to be the best version of myself I could possibly be. I feel incredibly lucky to have met her.

"She's going to leave you," says the imposter. "One day soon she'll realise what a fat, useless, pointless waste of space you are. And you'll be all alone again. As you should be." Its grip slowly tightens.

Imposter syndrome creates an incredibly toxic mental state. There is not treatment, no medication, no cure. It is both benign, and malignant; both passive, and aggressive. It has no externalities, no visible symptoms. But what it does do is plant a cancerous invader in your mind: doubt.

You doubt your abilities, your relationships, your very identity. Every aspect of your life becomes a battle to justify your own existence. To validate your place in the world. And what makes it worse is that you're not validating it to someone else, you're validating it to yourself.

And no matter what your loved ones say or do to reassure you, the imposter remains, whispering softly into your ear.

Gulls

Antosh, Writer

Time called to collect;
a Polish removal man
who twigs the surname.
It's all relative, eventually.
He begins with the lightweight
stuff; parts of Gran Gran
have risen to the ceiling,
a result of his recent, 'erosion'
hobby – smoking his appetite
out of the body, chain drawing
on a pack of twenty lighthouses,
waiting –
his means of controlling time,
keeping it marked.
The removal takes two packs.
House emptied, Gran Gran remains
below a fresco ceiling mural
of a new yellow – an ill sunset,
his fume marks hanging like gulls
do in paintings. He sits below
his designed sky, a lone,
heaviest matter, unwilling to rise
before the hunger, the turning
growl in the gut, has quietened.

Six years

Matt, Music Engineer

Six years…

Two thousand, two hundred and fifty eight days;

One hundred and ninety five million, one hundred and twenty three thousand, six hundred seconds.

It's funny, you don't realise that such a vast amount of time has passed until you really think about it like that. Nor how much a person can change in that time.

Six years…

The most significant thing that has happened in the last six years is being diagnosed with severe clinical depression caused by bullying; two six year cycles of teasing and plain nastiness all through my school years; psychological and physical abuse; teachers burying their heads in the sand. People pretending to be friends and then punching me in the stomach…

Six years…

I had just left uni and moved on to 'greener pastures'.

I was a different person back then, and I can remember then at the graduation ceremony looking back over the three years prior, thinking just how much I had grown as a person: how I had grown more confident, less afraid to trust, and feeling more self esteem.

I was terrified on my first day of university: terrified the same cycle of abuse would happen again from complete strangers. But it didn't. That fear ever lingered. But it didn't.

I suppose looking back now, especially now that double the time I spent in Uni has passed since I left, I was more naive than I could ever realised. Hindsight would have changed that.

Six years...

About half of that time I spent asleep. There were several moments I wanted to remain asleep because it was the closest to being dead I could get without actually physically doing the deed.

Many people were surprised with the diagnosis. I was not. "You are always smiling," "You exude such positivity," they'd say. No. It's a projection, or to quote lyrics from my music project 'Grown from Ashes', a false reflection of what I am actually feeling.

Inside, I was dead. I just didn't want close friends and family to know how much pain I was in. I just didn't want to be a burden. The blacker the darkness inside, the brighter I shone outside. We hide our pain.

Now I am on a diet of antidepressants and they have helped me ground myself. I am open as I can be after approaching suicide twice.

Six years...

I've lost friends – nearly all of my university friends actually. It's only natural. Everyone drifts apart.

Some of them I've had to cut out because their behaviours were toxic.

And I suppose, thanks to this, there are multiple things I've gained: wisdom; perspective. I have matured, I have thickened my skin.

I've gained a fiancée; a music engineering job; a life I feel is now worth living.

Life is a cycle of change.

I suppose the question is: what will the next six years bring? Who knows. Regardless, I'm here for the ride, however good or bad it gets. I'm ready to grow.

Grey

NWS, UK Student

When there's grey cloud above me
I feel no one will love me
I push everyone away

I resist this feeling, this storm inside
"Are you okay?" … "yes" I reply
Always knowing I'm being dishonest inside
Running away, ignoring it, trying my best to hide
"Are you sure?" always follows; nodding and smiling, I lie

But everyone knows how hard it is to pretend everything is
    alright
Soon you crack and everything goes black and then your chest
    becomes extremely tight,
gasping, not sleeping 'til the end of the night.

Sharp pains in your breathing
So far from healing
Self love has diminished and gone
Looking close and looking far, a continual feeling lingers,
like you never belong

To get away from the grey,
I hope and pray that things will be a lot better one day,
blue sky is my goal, sunshine to feel whole,
so I start meditating; mind, body and soul.

Telescope

Emma, UK student

he rinses his plate and
undoes the buttons of his shirt
showers and shaves
and gets into bed
as the ten o'clock news creeps up the stairs
he slots his shiny coin into the telescope
makes the most of his five minutes
looking over the sea

Park walks

Lily, UK student

The spring sunshine seemed to transform stern Glaswegian flats into beach houses. It took 10 minutes of my 30 minute allotted walk time to get to the park. I knew all the shortcuts. I spent a difficult 6 and a half months in this institution three years ago. I'd mapped every route to the park in my mind, the price of Diet Coke from each newsagent, where to walk to avoid the Christian conversion man, and the route each staff member took on their breaks and how to breathe normally if you were caught by one of them. Speed-walking, I could make it to the park in five. The park was always the end goal. Away from the staff, you could even jog if you weren't impartial to erratic pulse and serious scrutiny. Not worth it. Having stayed both 'voluntarily' and by law in several different institutions, I knew their systems. I had played the game both ways. Brutal honesty was at least truthful. One less thing they could hold against me.

This is the first time on my walks that I've forced myself to sit down. Half of me claps. The other half is less complimentary. I sit on the wooden bench with my legs crossed up underneath me, trying to ignore the pain already shooting through my body. Park benches are not forgiving on the bones. I force myself to stare at the horizon lined by tall city buildings and admit the day has been bearable so far. No breakdowns from anyone (yet). Nice weather meant the coffee trip went ahead and people can get out for walks. Heidi has time-out despite non-compliance. She is lucky enough to be under the same lenient doctor I had last time. I had to fight for this walk.

Two dogs circle around my bench. The first dog cocks his leg on the corner of the bench, narrowing avoiding me. I laugh in response. The owner, a tall man with dreadlocks, briefly scolds the dog. I pretend to look back at the city but I can feel the man's eyes on me. He says, "how long have you been here?"

It's a bold question. I know I don't have the strong Scottish accent, but I don't understand how he knows I'm not from here. Was it my laughter? I don't have the hearty sound of women born in the city. Did he catch the hint of sadness, the longing for home, within it? Perhaps it is because he is not from here either.

I am unsure how to respond. This stay; 6 months and counting. Hoping not to beat my record 6 and a half. Shortest stay: 4 months and a half at another institution.

"6 months," I tell him.

He frowns; "rough."

The dogs, bored with the bench and our conversation, continue walking past me, dragging their owner with them. This reminds me I've been sat down for too long, so I stand and start walking again even though my legs burn.

Candid

Becca, UK student

She doesn't see the camera,
doesn't know she's being filmed,
doesn't know she's standing there,
or anywhere. You might say

"The lights are on but no one's home," but
it's more like being trapped in
        a cupboard, deep behind her
eyes. She can hear the door-
bell ring, but she can only whisper
                messages for half-
deaf nerve cells to deliver. I watch

her try to smile. Once, twice, three
times, like she's casting a
spell to summon her-
              self. Some

ingredient is missing, some
component of a full per-
      son, locked in a glass case
or just out of reach from where she
is, down the uncanny valley,
so deep no one can hear her. I realise

I'm looking at a time traveler
seeing an invisible, prehistoric scene,
being very quiet, staying very still,
doing her best impression of a corpse
so the tigers leave her be. I watch

her, looking like she could glitch out
of existence any minute, and I think
"Oh. So that's what I look like."

A Letter to Ms Anxiety

BK, UK student

Dear Ms Anxiety,
In this surprisingly comfortable of unions
only you have the upper hand
while I play tug of war with my emotions
On those rare days when you'd unexpectedly bless me with your
  absence
I gather and still myself
Just like rain clouds do
just before the arrival of a fateful storm

The void

My body yearns for the healing touch of morning rays
But that was way back
before you came to bask in the winter sun with me
I let you cloud my rays with night shadows and bad tidings

The abyss

My tongue yearns for a taste of 'just' one drop of rainwater
I guess I never told you,
I used to stick my tongue out to catch raindrops
But that was way back
before you came dancing with me in the thunderstorm
I let us grow like wildflowers

The silence

In this invisible in-between life and death existence
You and I built a stone-walled tomb to seal this fatal union…

Untitled

Hannah, UK student

do you think Mother Nature knows about her children?
The ones that have been torn from her, born into tiny pots,
hidden from the sun and nutrients,
and barely allowed to grow at all.
forced to be usefully pretty,
before they wilt and die.
Maybe she's punishing us for what we do to them.

do you think Mother Nature knows about her children?
The ones that have been torn from her, born into tiny apartments,
hidden from the sun and nutrients,
and barely allowed to grow at all.
forced to be usefully pretty,
before they wilt and die.
Maybe she's trying to free us,
undo our separation

Immortal

Eden, UK student

Keyholes clogged with rust and scum
The slipway to my hidey hole harbour
Sanctuary from a waking world
Not long for this universe's judgment, or mine
Bear witness to the follies of allies
As the tally counter hits negative numbers
Heaps of mortals, life-expired
Those I enjoyed sharing a midday drink with
I'm here, waiting, watching the tumbledown door
As time's avalanche keeps sliding
Watch the sun die and the sky waver
As age aims and misses me again and again
Once more, twice shy, again and again
As my burning tonsils make me yearn death, again and again
I notice patterns in the creases and corners, again and again
I feel the floorboards giving way
As the scorched earth and aspirations poison and die
Nobody looked down, just out for themselves
Now not one has the grace to live on by me
Perhaps chance and luck will have its way with me
Court-ordered decision from beyond the grave for me
That I wasn't the survivor they craved, not me
I wish I could join you, wherever you are
Grant me relief, too little, too late
Again and again, again and again

Dressed in White

Inghild, Copywriter

Black grief is easy
to spot,
easy
to understand.
Not always easy to meet
but always
easy to accept

White grief
is not easy
to notice.
You're blinded
by the bright light
and your own
salutations.
You can't understand it,
you don't expect it,
so how
can you accept it?

ADHD Blues

Robert, Digital Marketing Manager

I was diagnosed with ADHD/ASD in 2013. Over the years, an exercise that fellow ADHD friends and therapists always recommended was to write a letter to my younger self, something I never made time for because of, funnily enough, ADHD.

Dear younger self,

You aren't feeling good about things right now. For as long as you can remember, you've felt like something was wrong, and 2012 was arguably the worst year of your life. If I remember correctly, you just wrapped up an editorial internship and played your first live performance with your new band, but despite many good times, you felt the opposite.

You've struggled with fitting in wherever you go, whether it's school, college or the workplace. That increasing feeling of anxiety and depression you have, sadly, you're still going to have it, but it's going to be much more manageable.

In your quietest moments, I know you get a sneaking feeling, an existential dread that maybe you weren't meeting your full potential. You have all the pieces of the puzzle but nowhere to put them. You need to know that you're going to get better. There will be a lot of work, conversations and medication involved, which will help, but having that diagnosis will bring a lot of understanding.

The next year you're going to do great. Just hang in there and remember that anything worth doing takes a little chaos. If I had to give you any words of wisdom or advice for the years ahead, just know that you're not behind. You're just where you are right now.

Best of luck,
Future you

Dead Weight

Ellie, administrator

He asks me why
I weep at home movies
and bawl my eyes out
on my birthday.
I shrug and walk away.
How can I explain that
I'm a promenading
graveyard?
That every moment
that is marked on
a calendar, stretched
upon a flimsy screen,
is just a lavish reminder
that I'm nothing
but a stain of time.
A revenant on
waking lands.
I dream of knocking
on the door of my
own casket,
I pace down sinking streets
counting my breaths,
I end every
conversation with a symphony,
just in case it is
my last.
I am a wreck of a woman,
always looking backwards,
always peering forwards.
When I realise that girls
my age cradle offspring,
I wish to purge poison.

When I get invited to ceremonies,
I cast out excuses to
cleanse my frontal cortex.
All I know is
I don't want to have
this hang up
my whole life
that makes me feel
as though I'm
carrying my
tombstone on
my back.
I just don't know
how to drop
the dead weight.

The Debt Unpaid

Catherine, Lecturer

The gritted path, the gritted teeth, the tip-tap of the pall bearers' Blakey's as they wobble under the weight of the boxed corpse and their own bloated guts, their grasping hands as blue as his are now. Top hats bob against the bruised pig-iron sky. The man with the duck's arse hairstyle leads the way with his black cane held aloft, a gold orb on a thin matt stick, a magician's wand, an extinguished lantern in the blank grey afternoon, shedding no light on the path to the 'under-the-ground'.

He's in satin. A modern shroud, Veronica had said. "All nice and cosy." They wouldn't let me see: "deterioration takes place rather quickly, and it *has* been two weeks since he passed away." Passed away. Passed to where? Hadn't he died? Wasn't I there? Hadn't I studied his chest? Didn't I count the slowing of the raspy inhalations while his throat constricted, his lungs wheezed, clicked and then terminally deflated like a punctured bagpipe? Didn't I wipe the sticky brown cloying mess from round his lips? Didn't I tell him I loved him? Didn't I lie? Well, did I?

Such a lovely man. So kind. Sadly missed. Sorry for your loss. We'll remember him so fondly.

"I love HER now."

Down in the hole, there are brown leaves, dead leaves, oak leaves. Brian picks up a frosted handful off the ground and chucks them in while we toss in red roses. Down he goes; down, he goes; down. He goes. The spell is broken. And after that, all I can do is walk away.

Rest, in peace

Tian, Digital Account Executive

I think of a soul
who wants to end their life
willingly
pleadingly
desperately.

I think of a soul
who looks into a mirror and
does not see
the mismatched edges
of their misconception,
who looks at the waterlogged white canvas
of their looming days
and sees drops of black
escalating
into gaping black holes.

There was never just one moment
of knowing
that there was no bluff to call,
that sharp metal objects
and volcanic water to the skin
were a prelude…
this infliction has been writhing
in the organs
raw
blood-soaked
primal,
volatile enough
to tear its way out
one day
into a fatal
crescendo.

I think of a soul
who wants nothing more
than to see
no more,
and I realise
that soul
is a lot like mine.

A painting of Human synergy

Polly, Humanistic Psychotherapeutic Counsellor

I try to paint a picture of human synergy.

With a heart that bears thousand scars,

I try to paint a picture of human synergy,

And I ask myself, am I too faint to paint?

Yet still I find a way to pick up a brush or maybe a lantern?

One more time,

To light the way for love,

A shot of dopamine! to motivate and be motivated.

Mental Health and Me

Emma, Recruitment Manager

Ill mental health
It started when I was young
Anxiety and depression
To my brain it clung.

Not understanding
Why I feel this way
Different emotions taking over me
Every single day.

Carbamazepine, fluoxetine, citalopram
Pills, just few of many
Why didn't my brain
Want to accept any.

Trying to block it out
Using self harm and drinking
Not registering that it doesn't help
And further you end up sinking.

As time goes on
It's like watching destruction
Unstable relationships, impulsiveness, dysregulation
It's one giant eruption.

I've had enough of everything
The crying, the pain, and the disassociation
I shouldn't be here
Is my realisation.

And then one day
Your loved ones worst fears come true
You overdose, trying to commit suicide
Because you can no longer be you.

When you awake in the hospital
People are crying
But all you can think is
I've failed, I can't believe I'm not dying.

Since then it's been a journey
A diagnosis of BPD
Emotional change doesn't happen overnight
But I'm trying my best to be happy.

Testing different therapies and coping mechanisms
Understanding not one size fits all
Relapsing for me is common
So I'm open with work, friends and family so they're there if I fall.

Today I feel lucky to be here
Even when life can be tough
But not every one feels that way
Look out for those who are feeling rough.

Reach out when you're concerned
Take note of the warning signs
Give them the hope
Of a lifeline.

Boys to Men

Pete, Digital Delivery Deputy Director

Growing up as a boy in rural Dorset, mental health was a bit like Latin – I knew it existed, but no-one I knew or could identify with knew much about it or took it seriously. It just wasn't for people like me.

Gradually at university and then at work I heard more about mental health. Friends would casually mention it was hard to get out of bed every morning or make jokes about how bad they were feeling with a laugh and a joke. No-one shared anything beyond that. I increasingly heard that suicide was the biggest killer of men under 50, and snippets of personal experiences of losing people. I wasn't particularly happy, and improving my mental health sounded like a bit of a silver bullet to make everything better, so I did some investigating. I read books on mindfulness and tried meditating, with no success. I self-diagnosed as suffering from Seasonal Affective Disorder (SAD) and then un-diagnosed myself when I still felt down in the summer. I even wrote a thesis on the impact of entrepreneurship programmes on the wellbeing of marginalised groups. But it felt like trying to learn and use Latin alone. It was confusing, not very useful, and a bit of a let-down compared to what I'd hoped for.

Reading an article comparing how mental and physical health are viewed and treated transformed how I thought about things. Gradually, I've realised that different things work for me at different times. Therapy has both helped and hindered me; talking to friends openly has been life-changingly positive, and excruciatingly embarrassing; giving myself a kick up the arse has reduced me to a dysfunctional mess and provided me with my best career experiences. I still can't meditate but I've found a few things that always seem to help. I ask myself if I'd ever be as hard on someone else as I am on myself. I cycle. I spend time with my son.

I've learnt to be sceptical of any solutions which are sold as solving everything, and to be more patient with myself and others. Talking about my mental health still doesn't come naturally to me but I'm determined to give my son the tools he'll need to thrive as a man, and that includes understanding and talking about mental health.

Empty chair

Georgia, Teacher

Over there an empty chair
The howls of laughter no more
Over there an empty chair
The warm embrace now cold to the core
Over there an empty chair
Ripped from beneath as she sat
Over there an empty chair
Not for jest, not for joke. Pain. Just that.
Over there an empty chair
How long should a soul's seat be filled?
Over there an empty chair
Only bittersweet memories not to be killed

Conquered? Catastrophised? Compartmentalised?

Luke, Teacher

These days I rarely cry.

I can't muster up the tears and then allow them to trickle down my cheeks. Does this mean I've conquered my ill mental health? Have I truly learned to not waste tears and channel my energy effectively, instead, into solving the problems that plague me?

Or, have I fallen even further down the rabbit hole? Am I in an even deeper, darker and emotionless state of depression? Perhaps it's one so nefarious that I've tricked myself into believing I've truly conquered the shadows that shroud me?

Perhaps I've achieved a stage of compartmentalism? Maybe I can place some woes and worries on the shelf for safe keeping – to be unpacked and played with at a later, or better, time. Meanwhile, when others arise throughout the day, could I be stronger and more prepared to tackle them to the point I hardly break a sweat?

Have I conquered?
Have I catastrophised?
Have I compartmentalised?

Surely the best answer would be a combination of all three?

To believe you've truly conquered ill mental health is an unhelpful utopia – and an incredibly foolish one at that. But to celebrate your achievements during your ill mental health journey is vital.

To constantly catastrophise will completely warp your sense of security and safety to the point of sheer – and devastating – hopelessness. Yet, a touch of tragedy never fails to shock the system and focus your mind on what's truly important.

To place all your troubles into tidy, organised boxes may cause you to build up a barricade to reality, dulling your senses from the flavours that life holds. However, this filing system of fears can allow you to tackle one trouble at a time and make that marathon seem much more achievable.

Maybe it's a healthy balance of the three. I conquer. I catastrophise. I compartmentalise. And that's why I feel the most in control of my mental health than I ever have before.

all my plants are dead

Katt, Artist/Lecturer

my doctor asked me how I was feeling
all my plants are dead
I said, hoping she'd know what I mean
she didn't

I wanted to invite my doctor to my house
to show her my dead plants but
I worried she would feel uncomfortable
in such an overpopulated graveyard

I would tell her that the dead plants
are metaphors for how I feel inside
my doctor would now understand
what I originally meant

I would ask my doctor to heal
my dead plants, maybe she
had a pill or syrup or something
my doctor would say,
nothing can save ~~you~~ them now

That Rug Really Tied the Room Together

James, ESL Teacher

When I was sixteen my family got a second dog. Buttons, a retriever, was getting old and tired. The idea was that getting a second dog would soften the blow when she inevitably died. So one afternoon my mother went out and returned with Fred – the runt of his litter and a mongrel combination of spaniel, terrier, and gremlin. He was entirely black, save a shock of white on his chest. He was a thief, a terrorist, and an escape artist. And then Buttons got her second wind and lived for another half decade.

As a puppy Fred slept in a cage in my bedroom, although the cage was an absurd charade. I was woken every morning by Fred jumping on my bed or shitting on the floor. Quite often I'd wake to find treasured possessions shredded like confetti.

The bedroom was large, with peeling off-white walls and a threadbare brown carpet that had been clumsily laid. The colour hid the stains. The ceilings were high, which meant a lot of wall space for posters. I had The Who, The Stones, and the Red Hot Chili Peppers. I was a big fan of the Chili Peppers, at least in the sense I had a Greatest Hits compilation I'd bought in Woolworths.

I stopped listening to RHCP after 2005. Partly because I grew out of them, but largely because of an unexpected visit from aunt that would turn out to be my first experience witnessing mental illness. It remains the worst, and easily the scariest and most scarring.

My aunt lived several hours away, and we weren't close. We saw her once or twice a year at most. Nobody expected her to knock on the door at 10pm on a weeknight.

By this point Fred was still a ball of energy and criminal tendencies, but he'd mastered bladder control and doing his business outside like a good boy. We'd put away the j cloths and stain remover, unaware all his hard work was about to be undone.

My aunt staggered in and started greeting us enthusiastically, as though she'd been invited and this was all perfectly lovely and normal. I assumed she was drunk, and just wanted to go to bed and read. Buttons was also disinterested, but Fred was overjoyed to make a new friend. He was thrilled to discover they shared a hobby.

The house had a long narrow hallway that turned out to be the perfect length and width for a rug my father had bought in Morocco. The rug was midnight blue and patterned with pink, green, and red flowers. It was a nice rug. Guests always admired the rug. *That's a nice rug* they'd say. *Oh, and it fits perfectly* they'd add.

Everyone except my aunt, who stumbled halfway down the hallway and then started urinating. Fred immediately and gleefully ran over and did the joined in. The rug was salvageable, but nobody could ever quite look at it the same way again.

My parents put my aunt in the kitchen, which had linoleum flooring. The kitchen had a little extension off to the side that contained, amongst other things, an old sofa and an empty birdcage. It was the furthest part of the house from the stairs, and also the easiest to wipe down.

I remember hiding on the stairs for a while, but at some point I was called down to fetch my personal CD player and some music. I thought my parents were trying to calm her down, but now realise they just didn't want her to overhear the phone calls they were about to make. I didn't own a lot of CDs, and most of what I did have was classic rock. My aunt smoked a soothing cigarette and chose the Chili Peppers compilation. Hard proof of an unsound mind...

When the mental health services arrived my aunt changed completely, and no longer showed any signs of erratic behaviour. There was nothing they could do, they said. And so they left.

As soon as the door closed behind them the erratic behaviour resumed. The police were called, because they didn't know how else to get her to leave, or get her help. They also feared her behaviour was drug related.

The arrival of the police more or less solved the problem, because the sight of them caused my aunt to become visibly erratic and she ended up kicking one of the officers. At this point the mental health services were called back, and she was sectioned – although I didn't know that, or what it meant, until much later. The rug was cleaned, the CD put away, and life returned to relative normality.

That night coloured my own perception of mental illness for a long time, to my own detriment, because my picture of a mental health episode was a picture of loud, violent behaviour and actually quite expensive rugs being micturated upon. I dismissed and downplayed other issues, and other people, because they were quiet, hidden away. Private crying rather than public urination. Behaviour that was irritating or frustrating but not wildly unusual. And often it's those suffering who hide or deny their problems, preferring to remain in a state of blissless ignorance.

I've learnt, over time, that for a lot of people their issues aren't always visible. Sometimes barely even perceptible. Sometimes mental health issues paint a picture bold and visible. Other times it paints a picture more like a magic eye puzzle, where you need really focus and squint at just the right angle to see it.

Buttons died in early 2009. I had just returned to university. I cried all day, and then got very drunk on very bad Korean lager. I watched *Terminator 2* and cried at the end. By the end of the week I'd dropped out of university. It wasn't until about 2019 I'd stepped far enough back to see the full picture for what it was.

Diagnosis

Eleni, Researcher

A rooster crows outside the window, ready to
reach for my throat. But I'm not worried about
his big teeth. I'm scared of the air around him.

He ruffles his feathers and becomes bigger.
He flies over the fence, escapes the barred
windows and people wearing daffodils.

No one else can see him, they all talk about the ants
running down my nerves, slowly eating my legs away.
The nurse plumps up my pillow, the TV shouts about

a dozen kids killed by a gunman in a city school.
But today, I don't care about their broken dreams
and unfinished homework, I want the results of my

tests, the dates for my scans. The doctor puts more
white pills in my palm. They look like the minty candies
we used to give to the beetles when we were kids.

We thought we could trick the beetles, tame them,
dry their lifeblood and put it in our school books.
We had courage and we had the tools. But they,

they had a pair of hidden wings and they had the air.
The rooster is outside the window, the nurse's hands
ruffle up the life chain, keeping me alive till tomorrow.

Own Worst Enemy

Lauren, Research Associate

I know how it feels
To be so locked inside yourself
That it's impossible to break free
To be strapped in a chair
While staring at an open door
To be the prisoner and the jailer
All at once
To have a body fighting to survive
And a mind trying to die
To be colourblind
Yet told constantly how colourful the world is
To be smiling on the outside
As you slowly fall apart on the inside
To be swimming in an ocean
With no land in sight
To have a perpetual shadow within
To be on a permanent losing streak
A master of breaking your own heart
Crippled with fear
Tormented by the demons in your head

So, let's just sit here side by side
And dry each other's tears
Learn to glide together
One step at a time
Until we can finally fly
Soar above the clouds
Seek solace in our shared distress
Live, not just survive

Alive

Amy, Content Writer

You are not a broken thing –
Made irreparable by the weight wrapped around your aching
   shoulders.

You may crack, splinter, crumble,
Even lose pieces of yourself,
Until you fear you resemble something unrecognisable.

But you are not a broken thing.

You are not drowning.
Though you swear you can taste the salt water in your lungs,
   choking out the last bubbles of air.

You may be buffered by the unrelenting, unforgiving tides until
   you are barely treading water.
But you are not drowning.

You are not lost.
Even if it seems you are stumbling blindly,
Hurtling towards uncertainty.

Tangled branches catching at you, ropes dragging you out of the
light, straying you from the path.

But you are not lost.

Broken, drowning, lost – you are not.
No, you are fighting. Surviving. One day thriving.

You are *alive.*

Food for the Soul

Johnathon, Software Developer

Last weekend you made a laksa. It was a poor imitation, but the most important thing about it was that it had a spoonful of peanut butter in it.

When you break up with someone – when you're broken up with – funny things tear the wound open. Weird things. Hot chocolate made on the stove, not in the microwave. A raven. Their name, written on the side of a bus, because God is real and she hates you.

Peanut butter.

You stare it and you remember the time you got a meal for free because the server assured you there were no nuts in the meal and then ran over screaming not to eat the bread. You think about the way they looked at you with pure shining love when you confidently told the takeaway place that nuts were absolutely forbidden.

You think about the way you stressed to your family that meals would need to be changed because anaphylactic shock would put a damper on any wedding, and then turned up without a date.

You eat toast with chocolate spread, or yoghurt, or you don't eat breakfast at all for a week. And then two weeks. And then six months.

It's weird, how habits form.

One day you buy a chocolate bar you've been craving for ages and then you bite into it and remember that when you had that chocolate bar before you spent the day being unable to kiss them.

They kissed you everywhere but your mouth and when you got home you scrubbed your teeth and swore before gods and men you'd forbid yourself from it forever rather than suffer another minute of being unable to kiss them.

And they laughed at your honest flamboyance and the way you wrap "I love you" in flowers.

You're suddenly not so peckish, but a bit of peanut sticks in your gum and bugs you the rest of the day.

And then suddenly one day this meal kit box you've got delivered – because asking yourself what you want to make is exhausting, because cooking is only a joy if you're doing it for other people – has something called a laksa in it. And the ingredients are laid out, and there's a little pot of peanut butter.

And your heart just sort of… thumps. Or maybe your ears work better. Or maybe you're inside your heart, somehow, staring up at cavernous walls and wondering how to get out.

And then you sort of… sigh. And you make it. And you taste it.

And it's the first time you've had peanut butter in 6 months.

And it's the first time I've had peanut butter in 6 months.

And it tastes salty, and my cheeks are wet, but overseasoning isn't the end of the world. And the next mouthful is better.

And the next is better again.

Little Voice

Alison, Recruitment Manager

I've always had this little voice,
Living inside my head.
It questions the things that I have done,
And judges the words I have said.
Little Voice makes me doubt myself,
It often tells me that I'm wrong.
This voice convinces me that I am not liked,
That I'm not like others, and I don't belong.
When things are going well,
It tells me that it will turn bad.
I can't tell anyone about this voice,
They will probably think that I'm mad.
I try to silence Little Voice,
To drown out the frequent sound and chatter.
But there are days when all it does is shout,
And that my sane thoughts do not matter.
I wish I was alone in my head,
Living this way is not a choice.
Instead my quest continues,
To tame my Little Voice.

Neverending Groundhog Day

Cat, part-time tutor

My mental health has been devastated by the intersection of two midlife menaces, the menopause transition and caring commitments, over 25 years for both parents. It impacts all aspects of life including work, finances, relationships and general wellbeing.

Carers are celebrated in national awareness days but for a lot of the time the responsibility and frustrations with systems that make up the daily challenges of caring leave us feeling very far from heroic and noble. Crying, shouting and ranting about the failures of medical, chemist, paid care agencies and hospital transport systems has led to my feeling of being in multiple halls of mirrors, with no seeming escape, going round and round in circles as everyone passes me on to someone else. 120 calls to get through to the GP, to ask where is the prescription that was ordered a week ago, is not an uncommon figure. Sometimes, most times, it leaves me breathless with tension and rage. My mind is no longer my own, hourly interruptions with parental misery or multiple professional queries blight my day and disrupt my capacity to think clearly.

In my imagination, my caring looks like holding my mother's hand, stroking her brow and singing songs from her childhood to her. In reality, it is more likely to look like rejecting my food or her shrieking at me to get out and leave her alone, despite the fact that she needs yet refuses help, and is often found on the floor after falls and illnesses. The force of will that kept her going as an abused child, now enables her to resist the increased frailty and its feared consequences. The fear and rage engendered by the later life combination of bereavements and memory losses, alongside ill health and constant pain, do not make for pleasant living, nor company. Life has become a seemingly never ending treadmill of appointments, complaints, parental suicidal expression, and institutional torments.

Stress, for example related to caring, causes changes in the endocrine system which knocks out the delicate balances that have been so hard won in relation to menopause, impacting oestrogen in the system and leading to increased brain meltdown and fog, panic, palpitations and extreme fatigue, accompanied by depression and lethargy. This in turn impacts my ability to hold down jobs requiring concentration, and limits my ability to carve out my own purposeful life. The financial worry that accompanies job insecurity leads round the stress cycle again to compound the distress.

Across 16 years, and many arguments and challenges to Doctors I have finally begun to get help for the menopause and feel much better. I am currently turning my lemons into lemonade and being a voice for those who continue to need support. Caring continues to be very difficult at times. And yet it will end one day, and then the sadness will change, mourning the better caring experience we might have shared, if only...

Big Up and Back Yourself

Esha, Senior Communications Officer

Do you ever feel like your sanity is hanging by a thread?
Like there's a huge battle going on inside your head?
And it's hard to explain, cause you feel so pathetic,
If you exposed how you felt, you'd surely regret it,

Would they think that I was weak?
Would they even care?
Am I self-aware or self-absorbed?

Did I open up or overshare?

Would they use it against me?
To belittle and berate me?
If after seeing me so vulnerable,
Would they ever take me seriously?

The root cause of my anxiety,
Is my lack of self-confidence,
The endless second-guessing,
And feeling like an inconvenience,

Self-analysing and self-abasing,
Self-destructive and self-critical,
I think I don't deserve good things,
And that's why I'm so cynical,

I don't try in case I fail,
I isolate myself from friends,
I sabotage relationships,
And make it a bitter end,

I dwell on my mistakes,
I'm convinced that I'm a villain,
I yearn for companionship,
But won't let anyone in,

My weight, just like my mood,
Forever fluctuates,
And the only thing I feed,
Is my growing self-hate,

Constantly feeling under threat,
And overwhelmed with regrets,
Replaying memories,
I'd much rather forget,

And fearing whatever,
And whoever,
comes next.

When I spiral out of control,
Darkness takes a hold,
I dig myself a hole, only to fall in,
And shatter into pieces below,

Can someone broken ever be whole?

And all it takes is one little trigger,
Did I sound stupid at work?
Is my stomach getting bigger?

I put the opinions of strangers,
Above what I think about myself,
Why be kind to everyone,
But be so cruel to yourself?

It's exhausting! It's draining!
I gotta get out this hole,
I have to break this cycle,
And take back control,

And I know just how to do it,
Cause it's been a long time coming,
It's time to face my fears,
Stop running, start climbing,

I'll build my self-esteem,
I'll be more empathetic,
I'll be more positive,
And less apologetic,

I'll be kinder to myself,
And braver, too,
Cause I deserve to be loved,
And so do you

Sickening

Lou, Content Manager

Sickening. A ripe fruit dripping venomous juice in my body, setting off scarred synapses with a SNAP – throwing me back to the past... or the present? I've lost it now.

"Tell me I'm safe. Tell me he's not coming, that he won't hurt me – tell me I don't deserve to be strangled and bruised."

Vulnerable words fall from my tongue, coated in that vile juice. A moment where scars are laid bare, ugly pink worms slashed across ribs, as fresh as the day nails clawed them into skin. A desperate hug, frail arms trying to hold it all together.

Breathe. It's been 3 or 4 years, or 120 therapy sessions? Welcome to the Now // the present.

Feel the floorboards beneath your toes. The home you've built on unsteady feet is stable enough to carry you through this, because this is just one moment of many that have passed since. A mash of memories led by neural pathways that are still being rewired. Say the words you need to hear:

"I am right now. I am right, now. // I am right here."

Notice how sweet they sound to your ear. Remember: Good mind, good body, good heart. Inhale, exhale. Each 5.5 seconds apart, until your unencumbered by what once was.

You are alive. Safe. Scared – but in no danger // free.

In 2016, you messaged me on WhatsApp.

A year later, I had to move my furniture to hide the hole you punched through my bedroom wall.

You told me I was crazy, that I was imagining things.

In 2018, you said you wished I were stronger.

You strangled me in a different city three days prior.

In 2019, we were at your dad's house and I lost my last straw.

My therapist said that with "neuroplasticity" we could fix my damaged neural pathways and rewire it to pass information along non-damaged ones.

Living with Mother

Fiona, Children's Librarian

I met a woman the other day who admitted that she had never felt depressed in her adult life. Unusual, we all thought. She then went on to explain that she thinks it was because her mother had a serious mental health problem and that she had grown up not knowing what her mother would get up to next. I can't tell some of the episodes she talked about as that is her story, but it rang a bell with me. My mother has a similar diagnosis and my brother and I from a very young age had an unusual upbringing. It wasn't easy having a Mother who one minute was a normal loving parent and the next was scaring us with her actions. I read a children's picture book recently about a child living with their mum who has bipolar. The author made it seem that there would always be someone else to turn to when mum wasn't well. This wasn't my reality at all. At first we thought our life was pretty normal but once we reached secondary school age it dawned on us that things at home were far from normal and that we had no one to turn to. As we grew older we often joked that we would reach the age of 30 and suddenly go mad like Mother. Well, we are now both well over the age of 30 and my brother and I have fared surprisingly well with our mental health and I can mostly say that I am probably more resilient than most. I'm thinking that I might go for a coffee with the woman I met who has never been depressed, so we can compare notes. I think it would be really interesting to hear a similar story from someone else's point of view and to probably congratulate each other on surviving our childhoods relatively unscathed by our experiences. As for that children's book, I'm sure the book would be reassuring to a child, if you had family and friends and other adults in your life to help, but if you don't, the reality of living with a parent with a mental health diagnosis, is very frightening, but may lead to you becoming a strong and resourceful adult. My brother and I and the lovely woman I met are testament to that.

Seeing life differently

Ed, peer support worker

I was first sectioned in a mental health hospital 20 years ago and in 13 years I was in hospital 14 times, it began to feel like my adult home. But I left hospital in 2016 and I've not been back, I guess I finally learnt how to live with schizophrenia and was mature enough to take responsibility for my own mental health. It took a long time to find the right medication and the right dose, but having medication that works is only the first step, feeling like a meaningful person takes empowerment and commitment. In the last 7 years I have built a strong life for myself, that includes working, writing, meditation, reading, sewing and exercise, I keep myself busy and have a very strict weekly routine. While my friends are getting married and having children, I'm busy writing my first philosophy book.

When I tell people I suffer with schizophrenia and episodes of psychosis they offer sympathy and say, well you're doing well now. The first book I wrote about my life was the first 4 years of my illness and I was a very angry young man. I worry that people will read it and think schizophrenia means violence and aggression, but that's how it was for me, everyone was telling me I was wrong and I hated it. As the illness progressed, I became more and more spiritually involved, earth, heaven and hell became real to me and my mission to save the world. But I became more isolated than aggressive, I settled down into the illusion and didn't need affirmation form the outside world. At one point I went looking for psychosis in street drugs, trying to find that sense of spiritual grandeur. Now I'm able to feel great without the immediate sense of saving the world, I'm a broken but beautiful person.

Looking at the world through the eyes of psychosis can be an incredibly revelatory process, facts with very little meaning, becomes signs of chance and fate. I have spent months fighting with demons and being loved by angels, but I wanted something more real, something that would connect me to other people's worlds. When I started volunteering I had very little work experience, but I slowly grew my skills and confidence, until I was ready for paid work and I've been in paid work for over 2 years. Using my experience as knowledge of recovery has given me grand ideas of helping all people with schizophrenia find work and meaning. I still get mini psychotic episodes, 'panic attacks' I call them and the medication makes me drowsy, I drink a lot of coffee, and sometimes I get the feeling of being incredibly special. But that's how my life is and that's how I like it, I've always thought of myself as someone who sees the world differently and I've always wanted to take an alternative path in life. Now I embrace my uniqueness.

The space in-between

Inma, Academic

You slipped into a region of fears
when you were trying to become yourself,
the landscape became obscure
and didn't feel safe.
Your senses always alert and raw
and you wondered
who you could trust in this strange world,
and you realised
no one, I am here alone.

Although we can't visit each other's land
because there are no visible roads,
we can still meet
in the sisterhood shores
swept by gentle waves of hope:
long embraces with our pressing hands,
shared meals, walks and games,
and touching cheeks and fleeting gazes
that know of fragility and love.

How to love your rot

Kate, Counsellor

I always knew I was angry, that was the easy bit.
It's easy to be angry when tears have been ignored, and needs
  neglected.
Anger was my fuel,
my fire,
my purpose.
I used it to push myself further and further.

From a child, isolated and alone that no one paid attention to. I
pushed myself, but it was never enough. I had awards, friends,
money, and I had fun. But something was missing.

Something was still rotting inside of me.

Every group I belonged to; I broke.

Insidious paranoia, feeling excluded, the attention I got was
never enough to fill the void inside of me. I realised that I didn't
know what love was. I built up a wall around me. A barrier so
high that it suffocated me. And that's when the break happened.
Finally, the last group broke, and I could no longer deny that I
was the problem. I had to think.

What am I doing wrong?
Who am I trying to be?
Who am I?

I realised I didn't have the answers, so I looked for them. I went
to a counsellor and talked.

I really talked.
And she listened.
To me.
Just me.

And I listened to me.

Until I had no more defences left. And that's when I cried. I stopped and I cried.

Behind the anger, locked in a pool of tears was my sadness. I was vulnerable, I was tired, and I was scared.

I always knew I was angry, but I never knew I was sad. It took me connecting with that sadness to find the rot. With my counsellor I took out my rot and examined it. And she didn't turn away. She held me, with my rot, and she helped me see that it wasn't my fault.

Until finally, I realised that it made me special, it made me who I am. In order to grow, I needed to look at my rot.

To love it.
To care for it.
Be kind to it.

And once I did that the anger felt more manageable, and the sadness less dire. My relationships improved.

I spoke to my parents about what had happened to me and found a language to explain how I was feeling to them. That's when I realised that they had their own anger and sadness

Their own rot.

I can't take their rot away from them, but I can understand where it comes from now and that it wasn't my fault, and it wasn't theirs. This experience changed my life, so I became a counsellor.

Because of my diverse upbringing I have empathy.
Because of the counselling I have a language.
So now I help others with how to love their rot.

The Winter Lady of the Dark

Sue, Unemployed

The Winter Lady of the Dark quivers,
It is the time of the owl, foxes hunt, squirrels sleep.
The seed in the womb snore, under an icy glaze.
Her dominion creeps out of a ratty's hole and sheltered places.
The core of the urban park in utter blackness,
Scratched with refractions of starlight on slithers of grass.

The Lady inhabits the cycles of the universe, she is the dark side
of the sun.
The Moon child, mistress of grief-scope, observing the
melancholy rooms of loneliness
Gathers Death's howl, as Innocence bleeds out of the holding
cradle.
She is demonic, Lilith, the unspeakable terror.
It is a journey of dark decay that call us all by name,
Galaxies to the smallest cells are subjected to her neutrality.

The Lady of Winter Dark is agitated, hounded out of urban
places,
Nestled in blackberry brambles, where rabbits braid her hair
and birds gather bedding.
She calls forth a bellow of furious storms. Resists the scent of
sweet spring shoots
Crackling her armour, gathering, creeping like tree-spiked
molasses
Ripping deeply into her membrane of existence.
She sinks with rocky tears into the mantle of Mother.

The Lady of Spring Light broadcasts in dank places her seeds to
    uncurl.
Faces lift up to the faint cries of promise,
And the park is dotted with sprigs of greenery,
Pregnant creatures sigh.
In the depth of the soil the Lady of Spring Light
Searches and tenderly drinks in her Sister's tears,
Merging like cojoined twins, one, yet always two.
Squirrels summoned to seek the acorn crack open the sky
And the oak of possibilities dances blindly towards the Lady of
    Summer Warm

Mental Ill Health

Thasky, Linguistics Assistant

Bang_Bang_Bang the call is unto us as men.
Bang_Bang_Bang the struggles we face each day are needed to be
communicated by us men.
Bang_Bang_Bang it will always take the best men to open his
chest and tell the truth about men challenges.
Here comes the booming sound of troubles and fear of a
syndrome called "what would people think of me, if I were to
confront my struggles as a man."

This is a disease that we don't want to confront.
This is a disease that we always sugar-coat it by day.
News flash, mental health illness knows nor age.
News flash, mental health illness knows nor colour.
News flash that mental health illness is befriended with
depression and anxiety.
News flash that mental health illness comfort zone is a graveyard.

We have seen greatest of men in South Africa committing suicide.
We have seen greatest of men declaring to be the quitters because
of this dreadful sickness.
We have seen priest turning into beasts.
We have seen teachers turning into thieves.
We have seen political leaders turning into Amaphara.
Oh well, we have seen it all through the needle in the haste.

Men are struggling to raise children because they are
untrustworthy.
Men are struggling to discipline children because they are
undisciplined themselves.
Men are struggling to take care of families because they are
unemployed,
Men are struggling to have the vision & mission of their daily
livelihoods because they are captured by the highest bidder.

The question is when this will stop so that men can have their essence of pride as men?

Without being patrilineal, men were once the head of the households but due to financial, emotional, spiritual, political, social, so-economic challenges men are just adding numbers to the communities not value.

Graveyards are full because men decided to be selfish, foolish and took their lives and leave children behind with a single mother.

Thanks to you Mental Health Illness for adding fuel to the fire.

Children are left behind as orphans because men decided to take the easy way out instead of seeking counselling.

Men need to understand that tears can help at times its okay to cry as opposed to the medieval notion of 'Ïndoda Ayikhali'.

In the world of triumph and disaster the only coping mechanism of man is alcohol.

This is a satanic stance that needs serious prayers so that men can pick up his manhood and follow righteousness.

We seek retrospection to men so that we can rebuilt our manhood and give hope to the young boys.

We seek role models so that men can talk more about mental health illness challenges.

We seek intervention so that men can have 'Men Imbizo' and speak about issue that are surrounding men (Mental Health Illness).

Glossary

Amaphara: South African term for the group of notorious young men who are capable to kill to get the next fix or drug. These young boys and men are at the age of 13-35, they feed their needs on methanol drug and they are addicts and jail birds.

Ïndoda Ayikhali: Literally mean men do not cry.

Can I have my life back please?

Andy, Unemployed

Can I have my life back please, I'm not finished yet,
There's so much more in life I want to see,
I'm just stuck at the crossroads, don't know which way to go,
Can someone come along and carry me,
Is it far too much to ask, to help me have a life,
To help me carry on and take the pain,
To somehow have a normal life, like everybody else,
Move forward, never looking back again,
See I can't see a future, I'm still stuck in the past,
Too many things that I just can't forget,
Things have really hurt me, and cut me up inside,
I'm still full of sorrow and regret,
See some things never go away, it's always on your mind,
Every time you close your eyes at night,
The flashbacks and the nightmares, they never seem to end,
Can somebody just stop it, make it right,
Maybe if I ruminate, and concentrate so deep,
I'll come up with the answers in the end,
Maybe give me therapy, and explain some things to me,
Maybe then my broken heart can mend,
See I'm still going over things, looking for a clue,
Looking for a reason for it all,
Was it my fault? Am I guilty? Am I the one to blame?
I didn't see it coming, dropped the ball,
Some people call it trauma, the things you cannot change,
All the painful feelings from the past,
I just want to put it all to bed, lock it all away,
Then I could have some happiness at last,
For others it is easy, don't dwell on painful things,
Pick yourself back up and dry your eyes,
It's easy when it isn't you, it's really no big deal,
Get over it, move on, forget the lies,

But they don't know the emptiness, they don't know how it feels,
When life it has no meaning anymore,
Left without the confidence, anxiety and fear,
No longer loving things that I adore,
Can someone give me choices, let me have some say,
Let me decide which way my life will go,
Hoping for a future, when things are not so tough,
Not frightened of the things I do not know,
See I'm not really guilty, for things that went before,
I didn't really ever have a choice,
I just want someone to listen, to what I have to say,
I'm still here and I've still got a voice,
I just need help to get there, it takes a little time,
It really is a struggle all the way,
But maybe if I stick with it and don't throw in the towel,
Tomorrow it can be a brighter day.

Winterish Thoughts

Anne, Retail Assistant

When winterish thoughts descend
I can feel like a leafless tree
Starkly silhouetted against ever-changing shades of grey
My bare branches stretched out to hold a place in the world
As roots burrow to anchor me from the wind's howl
There is nowhere to hide from this dark chill
Frost creeps under my bark
Silvered scars and knots of the past become visible
Vulnerable and exposed in this harsh glare I stand
All is etched into the rings of time
Sadness is shaped and held aloft
I breathe into my being and wait, wait
For a change of season, caresses of warmth
That bring bud burst and springs green relief

Rediscovery

Terry, Unemployed

You will smile again.
You will find joy in the smallest thing, again.

Healing

Bill, Mental Health Peer Support Worker

What's so amazing about the acronym CHIME?
That urges me to write this particular
Rhyme

A play on words for those in distress
This is my message for them to address

It just so happens, that we are much the same
All of us have been through our individual pain

No, it's not the physical type that I mean
But the pain in our brains that cannot be seen

Panicked into fear to cope with our plight
What shall we do?
Flight, Freeze or Face up and Fight

We try to discover the reasons of our sadness
When we're in despair they call it our madness

All that we want is answers, and for us to be heard
Understand our triggers and why they've occurred

Our painful pasts and the dreaded rumination
We must learn to relax and do mindful meditation

Fretful grim eyes with the frown on our brow
May gently disappear when in the here and now

The common ground that we all share
If we believe in ourselves in time will repair

We did not want it and certainly never chose this
This horrible thing that's described as psychosis

It's not our fault it might just be just our fate
Those feelings inside that we humans create

We will rescue ourselves from the fail in our lives
Just a small blip in our journey, we aim to revive

Do not think that this blip will last
That time won't remain
It's now in the past

We feel quite sour when our mind just curdles
We will learn to jump and leap over lives' hurdles

We must remain positive make life last long
Cherish each day and always remain strong

What is our destiny what is our role
Happy ever after this must be our goal

Do we know what reality is, or do we see it as virtual?
The truth might be found by being more spiritual

Looking for this we're all on the chase
Never look back hold onto this faith

Our inner strength it's part of our brilliance
We must never forget the power of our resilience

To find our holders of hope and no longer be sadder
We climb each step slowly to reach the top of our ladder

Scarred by anxieties and all of this depression
We will erase these marks with its stigma impression

Let's all Connect and always have Hope,
Find our Identity with this we will cope

When in doubt remember its Meaning
In time it will Empower us with a new kind of Healing

So, let's give a big thanks for all of this knowledge
That we have learned from the 'Recovery College'

Grateful thanks for your thought provoking gift
The pages of which we will reminisce and sift

Pathways to Recovery and "The Trail Is the Thing"
Will be our daily reminder and the joy it will bring

It's time to move on as we've covered the preps
We should now all be ready to take the 'Next Steps'

I will end this verse
As I started this Rhyme
I do find it amazing
This word that is CHIME!

Desert Dance

Rosanna, Disability Arts Facilitator

The oasis is yours
Every drop of water nectar
Every palm wave a caress
The locust cloud a symphony
The shimmering air your reverie
And you see the world in every grain of sand

The pooled water is your mirror
As you lean into yourself
You're dazzled by the miracle of your own reflections…

The Wild World calls
And with each footfall
The desert bursts with blooms of ecstasy

The sand dunes shift to surround you
No grounding, only shift, sound, light
You are dancing brightness, fire in flight
You are flame, you are furnace untamed
From flicker to inferno, back again
Inflamed by the dance, entranced by the symbols
Your steps make shapes like snakes across the sand

The gold sun held in your hand, the wind on your tongue

You are one with everything, everyone,
You sing with the sands
And dance Dust Devils
Spinning in sunlight delight
Not sensing the burn with the turning
The blistering skin, the glistening mirage
Soon to fade

And still you dance…

A fire that fierce burns fast to dust

Suddenly the sands shift to strangers, shrink away
And your feet sink deep

The wild is wilderness now
And you are... deserted

The singing sands sting your eyes, stick in your throat
You taste the dust and your thirst is endless
The desert is endless, pathless place
Every step is a scorpion
Lost in the vast and void, the worst is endless,
Nothing nears you, nothing hears you
And the beaming skies gleam cruel or careless

Every footfall opens an abyss, to move an inch is to stretch a mile
And when the storm comes in, you are lost... you are lost in
    dust...

Stormy seas

Rosie, Occupational Therapist

When the waves are crashing around you,
It's hard to take a breath,
When the sand moves from underneath your feat,
It's hard to stand up tall,
When your body feels like led,
It's hard to move out of the waves,

That's the moment when I remember the way the sun warms
    my back,
The beauty of wild water,
The feel of a strong embrace around me,
The refreshing smell of salt water,
The song that my grandpa used to sing,

I remember me,
And I take a breath

They saved me

Wayne, Mortgage Advisor

They'll never know what they did.

It's strange to think, of everyone I could have called or spoken
with,

It was the look in eyes of two dogs that saved me.

My Inner Child

Cometia, Swim Coach

I've been living with depression for most of life, but was officially diagnosis at age 38. At that time, I had simply checked out of life. I had been carrying a lot of trauma from my childhood, including abandonment, detachment, displacement, lack of nurturing, loneliness, isolation and the list goes on. Abusive relationships, and other disappointments also played a part in contributing towards my legacy of depression. I felt too weak to continue, what was the point as I was so unhappy. I placed blame on myself and couldn't find a way out of the dark place that was a prison in my mind. For some reason, I took full responsibility for the things that had happened to me, so I found a way to self-harm. I'm not sure if I really wanted to end my life, but I'm sure that I wanted to end the pain. I attributed all other failures in my life to something I had unwittingly done wrong in my past. My past, I call my Inner Child.

After all, my Inner Child is the child that is still suffering in my adult body. She cannot rest and will not allow me to forget her trauma. Even in my happy place, she reminds me that my happiness will be short lived, allowing negative thoughts to run wild in my mind, "you're rubbish", "you are nothing", "you are ugly", "no one wants you". When I am weak, I somehow feed these thoughts more, judging myself so harshly that it's almost impossible to get out of bed, brush my teeth, eat or face the world. Somehow feeling like the outside world knows and will be judging me also.

After months of hiding, not eating, not drinking, laying down in the same place looking like a bag of bones, my friends staged an intervention and along came the psychiatrists, counsellors, therapists, and doctors. All trying to keep me from checking out of life. I didn't want to exist, because to exist meant that I will still have to deal with the problems in my head, in my memory.

I refused to talk to these professionals. Why where they in my life, why did they care, I did not ask for help, I was not bleeding, I was not sick. I was just extremely sad. This is not an illness, I argued. I didn't want to take up the professionals' time, I wanted them to treat real patients, real pain, not my sadness. I felt guilty for taking up their time. They couldn't make things good in my head, they couldn't take away my painful memories or erase my past. But they convinced me that I have depression and this was indeed an illness.

Today, with cognitive behavioural therapy through MIND charity, I am living with and managing my depression. I wish I could say that I am depress-free, but I realised that I will never be free of this, so recognising what triggers it, applying my coping strategies, and enforcing my structured routine. I do have the odd relapse now and then and always resort back to the comfort and safety of my bed, cover my head and ignore the world.

My counsellor's parting words to me: "I'm afraid that one day you will wake up an 80-year-old woman, having not lived your life, as you are allowing your past to dictate your present. You are in charge of your life now, so put your Inner Child to sleep, and go forth and live your life."

What does resilience mean?

Kath, Digital Strategy Lead

What does resilience mean?

"We need to learn resilience Jack."
"What does resilience mean Granny?"
"It means expecting the best, and then accepting what comes."

This was a conversation between my mum and my eldest child in early 2012. Jack was having a tantrum because the roundabout wasn't working, but I suspect mum was thinking about something else – she was looking after 4-year-old Jack because I was in hospital with Alex, his 9-month-old brother, who had just been diagnosed with an aggressive cancer in his skull and had a 60% chance of survival.

11 years later, we still talk about resilience lots – but we also recognise that nobody can be resilient all the time. Alex has a much better chance of living a long and good life. He is blind and has a brain injury as a result of his tumour and gruelling year of treatment, but he's officially in remission which is wonderful. He is funny, talented, eloquent, and worries about lots of things. Jack is 15, strong, bright, opinionated, kind, and at times very anxious and sad.

I co-parent the two children with their dad, we get on well now after separating 7 years ago. We inexpertly juggle work, parenting and other commitments. We both have days where we think we just can't manage. I realised recently that the trauma of the last 11 years has taken its toll – I cry easily, I'm anxious, I don't sleep well, I have developed some bad habits to try to cope, and I sometimes find myself on the brink of collapse. I've got better at recognising when that is happening and taking steps to recover – mostly that means being calm, resting, stopping doing so much stuff, being on my own, walking, breathing, sleeping.

Resilience comes from gratitude (says my friend Anja, a leadership coach). I didn't understand but now I do, I think – you can weather any storm if you genuinely feel grateful for your lot. And we can learn gratitude. That doesn't mean pretending that nothing bad happens, being relentlessly positive and sweeping everything else under the carpet (although I have a tendency to do that sometimes). It does mean spending a bit of time working out what you're grateful for, and celebrating that.

I sat with the children in that time between Christmas and New Year – my time to have a clear out (my messy house, my messy head). We wrote down the good things about 2022, the things we were proud of, the things we enjoyed – and the things we wanted to chuck in the bin (Jack's was "mean people being mean" and Alex's "rollercoasters" – slightly inexplicably as he has never been on one). Then we thought about what we wanted to do more of next year. "Play with my toys, but no rollercoasters" (Alex). "Play music and do drama" (Jack). "Spend more time seeing friends I love" (me). It's good to have achievable aims.

We are working through the impact of the last 11 years, with the help of friends, family, and lots of incredible health professionals – I'm hugely grateful for the support we have, which helps us to be more resilient, enjoy the good bits and muddle through the less good bits. I try to keep Mum's mantra in mind – expect the best, and accept what comes.

Wordsmith

Stephan, Poet/Writer

My therapist tells me I need to be more honest with people.
When the voices in my head prickle under my skin,
syllables imprinted across my eyelids
and slamming against my skull;
it's harder to escape nightmares when you're awake.
I say I'm okay because it's easier to pretend
and I've always liked being someone other than myself.
Do you know what it's like to hate yourself?
To despise every word that falls from your failed lips,
each letter smashing on the ground when no one reaches to
    catch them
and you try to piece them back together
but the glue is hot and acrid and suddenly you find it hard to
    breathe
as your fingertips melt away
and your teeth trickle to the floor
and you don't know who you are anymore.
I say I'm okay because I haven't hurt myself this week
even when the cravings coated my tongue
and made it impossible for me to speak.
I spend hours in the shower,
skin hissing under scalding water
as I scrub myself raw even though
I will never truly be clean.
I say I'm okay because recovery and relapse mean the same
    thing
and does it even count as a relapse if I never stopped?
It's easier to lie because lying keeps people in the dark
and the truth looks too ugly with a spotlight shining on it,
exposing truths so bitter
it feels like you're wearing a barbed-wire scarf.
Each time I try to speak, try to shout, try to beg for help –

I am drowned out, shame smashing over me like high tide
and I want to hide away,
find a shell to slink in to and live like the hermits,
nothing but sea glass and mottled rocks and sand blankets.
My therapist tells me I need to be more honest with people.
My therapist is a fucking idiot.

Be Like Them

Hannah, Lecturer in User Lead Research

I've been staring at the ground so long I've barely seen
The cracks in the blue sky that the clouds were moving in.
These buildings that had me trapped,
Their crumbling walls ain't even attached.

I've tried to live my life but I've done it so small,
Tried to copy others leaping when I could barely crawl.
I will never be the same, I think, as I watch them dance
Like shells moving with the tide in their trance,
Easily, instinctively, blossoming from the day they were seeds
Whilst I, stilted, frigid, shrunken and frozen in the weeds.

The places they'll travel and they things they'll see,
All the light they'll grow in places depression has never been.
So I boarded that plane, I was destined to find
A high so high, with all of life unravelling through their eyes.
A human doing what the beings said it should,
But I never made it to their forest for the heaviness of the wood,
Stick legs trying to run through mud,
Falling heavy, abandoned with a thud.

I just wanted to run like them,
To run at speed,
Dance their dance
Know how to be free.
Get drunk and follow,
Towards the stream,
Tiny pieces,
Of us that gleam.
To box what is broken,
Embrace changes,
Thoughts that sting
And empty strangers.

To be a child of wonder,
Collecting shells on the beach,
Tumbling Lego walls,
Into the breach.
To give up all fight,
Things let be,
To know hope
In all its permanency.

The Kindness of Strangers

Alan, Service Delivery and Transition Manager

Talking about your feelings, telling people how you actually feel, it's not a man thing is it? It certainly wasn't when I was growing up, either at home or with my friends. You had a problem, you bottled it up, and just hoped it went away or sorted itself out!

I lived about 35 years on this planet believing this was the right way to do things, that telling people about things that were worrying me just wasn't the socially acceptable way to conduct myself. "Be a man" I'd tell myself, or the phrase that now boils my blood "Man up"!!

It was in my 35th year that I went through a bad relationship break up, my home life was destroyed, my work suffered, my children suffered, I had no-one I could really talk to, everything just got too much. That was the first time I had any dealings with a Mental Health First Aider (MHFA). After many failed attempts I finally plucked up the courage one day and reached out, one of the reasons I was scared was that I thought my problem was trivial in the grand scheme of things, there's people with a lot worse going on who aren't falling to pieces so why should anyone care about my silly break up worries?

I couldn't have been more wrong. Telling a kind, caring complete stranger all of my fears, worries and anxieties was like a light switch turning on! How did I ever think it was ok to keep it all in, to live with the burden all to myself, when there are actually people I work with, who volunteer their own time and have been trained to listen and help their colleagues.

Sadly, after this interaction all of my problems weren't fixed, they didn't just go away, but I felt lighter, I felt like I could breathe again, and I felt forever grateful to that stranger who had taken the time to listen to me, without any judgement, and they signposted me to the people who really could make a difference to what I was going through.

6 months later I volunteered to train as a MHFA, the help I had received forever ingrained in me and I was looking to pay that forward in any way I could. They are just normal people; they are your colleagues and friends who sacrifice their own time just to listen. They do it for free, above and beyond their day job, simply because they want to help.

Talking to a stranger really can change your life, I should know. Nothing is ever as bad as you imagine in the depths of your own mind. Reach out, please.

A man called Harry

Little Em, Granddaughter

When he was…

When he was young, he was an orphan
When he was old, he was surrounded by family
When he was young, he was striking
When he was old, he was devoted
When he was young, he joined the navy
When he was old, he played golf
When he was young, he got married
When he was old, he taught his grandchildren
When he was young, he cared for others
When he was old, we cared for him
When he was young, I didn't know him
When he was old, I knew him inside out
When he was young, he could've lived forever
When he was old, he died in my arms
When he was young, he was known as Harry
When he was old, he was known as Ace
When I was young, he was my everything
When I am old, I will remember him, always.

Writing on a stone

Alun, Head of Student Life

It's hard isn't it to say how you feel
It's hard to articulate a thought and share
It's hard to be to be who you expect to be or live to the
     standards you set
It's hard when everyone seems to be more put together
It's hard to send that help email
It's even harder to hide how it all feels
It's even harder to deal with all the things you have built pretty
     epic compartments for
It's even harder to keep routine or stay motivated
But
It's impossible to keep going like you are
It's impossible to hide it forever
It's impossible to keep the tears back
It's impossible to cope unless you admit it
Admit that you're a human
Admit that being a shoulder to cry on doesn't take it's toll
Admit that it gets too much sometimes
Admit that sitting in the car for an extra five mins is alright
Admit that staying on top is keeping yourself in check
Be strong
Be hard
Be a man
Be a lad
Be whoever you want to be
Just don't be a name on a stone

Recovery

Sanjeev, Retired

Being in the presence of the people I love,
Watching their love,
Feeling their love,
Gives me the energy I need to
Recharge
Reset
Relook
At the way I view my future.

My Story

Chris, Business Partner

Ever since I was a child I have always been anxious or nervous. It did not effect my normal day to day life, but this began to change when I was in my early 20s.

The first time it did start to affect me I started to have panic attacks. This was about the same time that I had developed some food allergies, and my first panic attack was the day after I had an allergic reaction. At first I thought that it was another allergic reaction and an ambulance was called, but it soon became obvious that it wasn't.

After this first panic attack I started to have them quiet regularly for the next few weeks. I was probably having around 3 per week and it was really taking it our on my both physically and mentally. This is when I started to take medication, but it took a while for it to kick in.

One of the worst panic attacks that I had at the time was at a train station in Twickenham after watching England play Rugby. The train station was completely full and you couldn't move. This is when I started having a panic attack and couldn't get on to the train. This is the first time that my friends have seen this happen to me, and some of them were not as understanding as I expected. I was surprised though that when some of my friends were not understanding of the situation, the rest of the group stood up and helped me through the situation.

After this I started to try putting in some coping mechanisms in place, things such as breathing techniques and not drinking or eating sugary things. I found that this was one of the things that caused me the most issues. I would find that if I had had a lot of sugar then this would mean I would have a panic attack later in the day.

Fast forward a few years and I had really got my anxiety under control. I had stopped taking my medication and I hadn't had a panic attack for years. Then COVID happened. All through the summer and autumn I was fine, but then as soon as winter hit it really started to affect me. It all started because there was a huge amount of time where I would not leave the house, and then when I did I was having a huge number of panic attacks and crippling pain and sickness which lasted for months. I was unable to go to the shops, take the kids to the park on my own. The only way I could go out and feel comfortable was with my wife, but even with her, unless I was at a friends/family members house it was a real struggle.

This went on for around 8 months. In this time, we sold our house and brought a new one, and it made it very difficult to view homes because of the panic attacks. There were a number of times that I would have to cancel appointments because I was unable to get out of the car. I very quickly went back on my medication, and it took a while for me to restabilise and get back to where I was before. If I am being honest I probably still am not back to my best but I am well on my way.

I would not have been able to get through all of this without my wife and kids, family and my friends at home and at work.

Intrusive

Tom, Library Assistant

I thought you were me.

For so long, I thought you were me.

Whispering things I didn't want to hear, showing me things I hated to see, moulding me into someone I didn't want to be.

For so long, I thought you were me.

But you're not me.

You're you.

You're you and I'm me.

It was a word that made me realise who you were. A word, staring at me on a computer screen.

Intrusive.

It brings to me so many other words. Unwelcome. Uninvited. Invasive.

Invasive.

I woke up my soon-to-be-wife. It was early morning but I hadn't slept. I hadn't slept because of the thoughts and the actions I had to do because of the thoughts.

I woke her and she asked what was wrong.

I told her I know what I have.

I know what's wrong with me.

I know that this is not me.

The doctor made more sense of it all. I spoke about the thoughts, though not in detail. Just enough. She nodded, scribbled down notes and made humming sounds. I worried she'd turn me away. Say I wasn't getting enough sleep. Say I spend too much time on my phone. Tell me this is something we all go through.

On the other hand, I was worried she'd believe me.

I was worried she'd suggest locking me up. She'd suggest I was unsafe. She'd suggest an intense, psychological 'fix' of me.

But that was you saying that, wasn't it?

That was you.

You wanted to live in there, continuing your poisoning unchecked.

The doctor gave me a leaflet. A diagnosis. Three letters. I thought I'd hate to hear them. But I didn't. I loved hearing them. Because now you had a name.

You're not gone.

You don't disappear.

Even with the therapy, even with the medicine, even with the wonderful things that have happened to me.

You're not gone.

And you're not me. But you're part of me. And I can manage.

Letters

AM, Teacher

12.41 am   30/10/2022

It's been an emotional evening and I wish you had been there with me. Telling my best friends about you only confirmed what I already knew, that it's you. It's always been you. Before I even knew you existed. I was loving you. In every dating app, in every heartbreak, and in every tear I would sob wondering why I couldn't be what someone wanted. Every day you are healing my scars a little bit more, and every day my guard comes down a little lower. Every day makes me realise that I won't ever want this to end. So let's face love together, because I only want to feel it with you.

Always us.

10:47 pm   09/11/2022

5 weeks ago today, unknowingly, our lives took a turn. Or maybe it wasn't as unknowingly as I thought. Because I knew after that practise that I wanted to find a way to start a conversation with you. I think my heart knew it was you before my mind could even begin to accept it. I wasn't ready to accept my life might not look exactly how I imagined it. And over the past 5 weeks, I've tried my best to accept what is going on. While I'm not embarrassed, ashamed or disappointed, there's still the expectations of others that have been placed on me. And I am sure one day I'll accept it finally to the rest of the world. Right now, I accept you, and us, and the most incredible magic we share. You are everything I've ever wanted. You are kind, and smart, you're attentive and oh so loving, and the most beautiful girl I've ever laid my eyes on. You're my confidant and my comfort blanket. The keeper of my secrets and the sharer of my world. I love doing life with you and I hope it never ends.

All my love.

The link between physical and mental health

Katie, Delivery Manager

Thank you to my Doctor.

You listened.

You didn't give up.
You believed me without hesitation or questions.

You put me first.
Me, as a whole person, not just a person with pain.

You truly helped.

Never underestimate the power of persisting and asking for the
help you deserve.

The anxiety of "What if"

Laura, Civil Servant

I worry. I worry every single day. I worry about worrying.
Worrying is like an endless ball of knotted string.
You can never see the end, it is buried inside.
Some days you can't unpick the first knot and other days you
    unpick knots all day long.

I worry. I worry every single day. I worry about worrying.
The words "what if" have become part of my daily thoughts
What if… I'm not a good enough friend
What if… I'm not good enough at work
What if this happens… what if that happens… ?
I worry. I worry every single day. I worry about worrying.
The "What ifs" become a ball of string in their own right
At the end of the day, I can end up with a bag full of strings
A bag full of strings that I have no use for and I can't re-use
Tomorrow is a new day, with a new ball of string
I worry. I worry every single day. I worry about worrying.
I worry that I'm worrying too much. So much, that it makes me
    worry more.
It's easy to say "don't worry about it" but it doesn't help me stop.
I say I'm a born worrier, because I don't know anything different.
I know worrying doesn't help, but I can't make it end.

A Haiku for Hope(lessness)

Glenn, University Associate Dean

I wasted my youth
Wishing tomorrow would be
Better than today

I didn't realise I didn't have to hate myself

Jen, Head of Design

I didn't realise I didn't have to hate myself.

I've always grown up hating myself. I didn't know any different – I think I thought everyone did. I once made a list of all the things I hated about myself and it pretty much included every single thing about me, with the exception of my nose (for some reason I was fine with that). A friend of mine found it and was really upset by it. She couldn't imagine why I'd do that to myself. But I didn't feel like I had a choice.

You wouldn't ever know this about me on the surface, of course.

Over the years I'd occasionally be overcome with the feeling and need to just withdraw for a few days. I'd get over it and go back to being ok on the surface.

Life goes on, and you do your best to cope, but it still happens. My husband has a mental health condition that nearly knocked us all over at one point, but we coped. A couple of years ago, my son was diagnosed with autism. And something happened that took me by surprise – we were rejected by many of those around us. He "needed to move schools", we "weren't being good parents", or were "just using autism to cover up bad behaviour". My anxiety went through the roof and I badly wanted to take to my bed. But I had a feeling that if I did that I would never get back out again. I didn't leave the house for a month (though on my work calls you probably wouldn't have known).

I did something I hadn't done before – even in my self-loathing, I asked for help. I started with talking therapy but my GP suggested I also try antidepressants. I hadn't wanted to previously (or was it that I didn't like myself enough to help myself?) But doing both together, slowly, I felt stronger. That was 18 months ago. A couple of months ago, I was sitting, drinking coffee, and I realised – I don't hate myself. I thought of that young girl with the list and wished I could have told her she could cross things off. There are things I don't like, but I see them either as things I can work on or things that just make me who I am.

That's not to say I'll always feel this way, but it's been so lovely to give myself a break.

It Gets Better

Ryan, Charity Worker

Feeling like a stone rolling down a hill
Like an empty cup you're unable to fill
Feeling hollow, numb, in a pit of despair
Will it ever get better? Oh, I have been there.

It gets better.

It may not feel like it now, it may be a while away,
But hope is not lost, there will come a day
When it gets better.

And I tell you, when that day comes,
The end of the battle that you have won,
You'll feel a calmness, a sense of relief,
Confusion, Conflicted and disbelief.

A realisation that a chapter's at its end
At least for this moment, you'll feel you again.
Another page turns in your story of life
You'll be that bit stronger, overcoming that strife.

And yes it may be that dark days will return
But you can look back at these times
Take comfort from what you have learned
Take a breath,

It gets better.

Family

Julie, Head of Office

I was about 7 or 8 when I realised Mum was different. She would spend her days in bed or sitting in a chair in our living room drinking endless cups of coffee. She never spoke – just stared out of the French windows with the dog by her feet.

As a family our basic needs were met – our clothes were clean and we were fed. The meals we had were simple and now I am an adult I realise that we lived on a tight budget. There was little or no interaction with my Mum – she was just there in the house – but that was what it was like for everyone right? It wasn't until I was invited to other friends' homes for tea that I realised things at home were at the best dysfunctional.

Mum suffered Postpartum psychosis after I was born. She was very unwell and subsequently resulted in several months stay in a mental institution and my maternal grandmother who lived 100 miles away raising me for my first 6 months of life. Of course, I have no recollection of this but suffice to say when dealing with my own mental health it transpires that I didn't make the connections I needed to with my Mum as I was separated from her.

This was the 1960's mental health care was in its infancy and there were limited treatments. After drug therapy was exhausted, electroconvulsive therapy (ECT) was tried – this is where the patient receives an electric current to their brain through electrodes placed on the head. I shudder at the thought and from what Mum can recollect of this she found it unpleasant and unhelpful.

My sister arrived 3 years after me – the doctors thought she may swing Mum's mood back to normal and whilst things didn't get worse – they didn't get any better.

By now Mum was suffering from psychosis – she would see things and hear noises (usually voices) that weren't there.

I guess by now you were wondering what my Dad was doing? He and Mum had moved to Coventry in the early 1960's as part of the economic boom in the city. They left their friends and families in north Wales/Cheshire. Dad was trying to keep down a job and raise 2 kids in effect. In addition to this he would take Mum to her mental health day care – we were passed around friends regularly. He struggled for many years trying to make it all work and just after my 18 birthday he left and has never looked back. The chains of Mum's mental health have been picked up by my sister and me. We have had to make some difficult decisions over the years.

My Mum's head is still in the 1960's, she has never been able to hold down a job, the treatments she has had have meant she has cognitive impairments. As a family (my sister and I) we have to manage everything for her from her housing arrangements to optician appointments. She gets easily confused and will often make up stories where she has gaps of missing information – which makes it hard to understand what is real. She still hears voices and sometimes sees people – particularly those who are no longer with us.

My own mental health has been affected over the years, my health visitor recognised signs of postnatal depression after the birth of my first child and sensitively guided me to my GP who was amazing. My depression has stayed with me throughout most of my life and when it gets tough, I will engage in talking therapies. At 57 I still take antidepressants as without them I struggle.

Perhaps the saddest thing is we have no mother/daughter relationship so there is nothing to talk about in any depth. She has a superficial interest in my children and has had very limited input to their lives. Unfortunately, her illness makes her focus on her needs only.

For me this is the Mum I have always known – I mourn the loss of a relationship that her mental illness took away, I mourn the fact she cannot help me when I am down, and I mourn the life she has lost to her mental health. I feel it is my duty to care for her and I admit there are days when I would rather not. Does that make me a bad person?

I am lucky: lessons from a social worker

Vita, Programme Manager

I feel lucky.

For all my life, I've been used to talking about mental health. I was brought up in a household with a dad as a social worker. My gran was a social worker.

I feel lucky.

They taught me to focus on the things that made me feel well and encouraged me to focus on the important things: family, friends and fun.

I feel lucky.

In difficult times, I was given the space to talk and explore difficulties.

I feel lucky.

Even though, at the time, they didn't know the science, they promoted their worldview that mental and physical health were intrinsically linked. I keep my body healthy.

I feel lucky.

They surrounded me with love and support. I surround myself with people who champion me, and I give all I can back.

I feel lucky.

They reminded me that challenges are relative. This didn't mean that certain difficulties were less valid. They taught me to keep perspective and to remind myself...

I am lucky.

We can't go back

Ella, Communications Assistant

And in some ways I'm thankful.
And in some ways I wish I saved myself.
From the trauma of a brain gone wrong.
But I know I would be a different person.
Time is linear but I'm counting down the seconds back to
    where it all started.

And who doesn't like a recovery story?

www.ingramcontent.com/pod-product-compliance
Lightning Source LLC
Chambersburg PA
CBHW041732200326
41518CB00019B/2576